Sex and ♂ Relationship ♀ Education

The no-nonsense resource for sex education in primary schools

FOR AGES 7–9

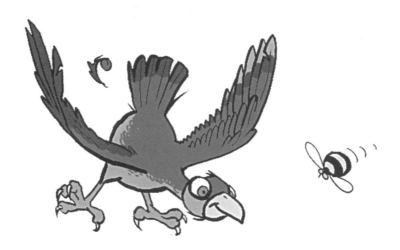

MOLLY POTTER

This book is dedicated to Suki Dell – for all

that she has taught me – with such

enthusiasm and patience!

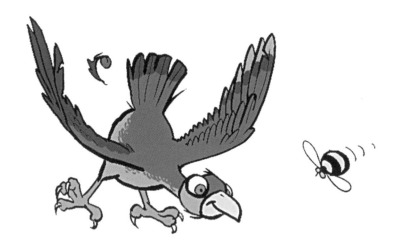

First published 2009 by A&C Black Publishers Limited
36 Soho Square, London W1D 3QY
www.acblack.com

ISBN 978-1-4081-1069-0

Copyright © Molly Potter 2009

Written by Molly Potter
Design by Anita Ruddell
Illustrations by Mike Phillips/Beehive

Printed in Great Britain by Martins the Printers, Berick-upon-Tweed

This book is produced using paper that is made from wood grown in managed, sustainable forests. It is natural, renewable and recyclable. The logging and manufacturing processes conform to the environmental regulations of the country of origin.

To see our full range of titles
visit www.acblack.com

Contents

Introduction

The key messages that help schools to feel positive and more comfortable about their Sex and Relationship Education (SRE) can be summed up in a few bullet points:

★ There is a lot of anxiety about SRE. Much of the anxiety comes from our own (usually) less than favourable experiences of learning about sex and body parts, and this can be addressed.

★ There are effective 'tools' of good practice that can help everyone to feel more comfortable in SRE lessons.

★ Most parents/carers are supportive of the SRE schools deliver to their children.

★ SRE is embedded in the Personal, Social and Health Education (PSHE) curriculum and, although teachers often cite that they need most support with delivering the biological aspects of SRE, the non-biological aspects are far more likely to have an impact on the decisions children and young people make than factual knowledge about sex.

★ A significant part of SRE is about equipping children and young people to protect themselves. The information they gain from SRE does not 'damage' them if taught sensitively.

★ Children and young people live in a world where the media and other sources bombard them with often 'unhealthy' information about sex, body image, gender and relationships. One of the aims of effective SRE is to give children and young people a more balanced and realistic view of the world in terms of self-image, sex and relationships.

★ Research shows that nearly every adult who shows some level of resistance to their children being taught SRE can be made to feel completely comfortable with this issue when the right information is disseminated.

> **IMPORTANT NOTE**
> SRE programmes vary from school to school. Some schools would be happy to use all the materials in this book whilst others may deliver less comprehensive programmes. It is up to each individual school to devise a programme that it believes suits its pupils.

So what is this book?

This book is a complete package of materials that can be used to devise and support your school's SRE programme and policy. Not only does it include curriculum materials, it also has resources that can be used with parents/carers, school staff, governors and pupils to help everyone 'buy into' the idea of an effective SRE programme.

What's on the CD?

★ Printable documents of the entire book.
★ Editable versions of selected activity sheets and information pages which are indicated by an *.

How is this book organised?

This book is split into three sections:

★ Useful information, documents and training activities to help support the whole school involvement in programme and policy development.
★ Activities, lesson plans and photocopiable sheets from which an SRE programme can be devised.

★ Appendices — forms and letters to support SRE development.

Why does this book contain so much biology?

SRE in its full definition makes up a large part of Personal, Social and Health Education (PSHE). However, when schools ask for help with SRE, they are usually asking for support with delivering the 'sex bits'. Schools are generally comfortable delivering the PSHE or 'relationships' component of SRE.

How can the curriculum materials in this book be used?

Many junior schools have started to realise that teaching SRE in the last half term of Year 6 is too little and too late — especially with respect to covering the changes of puberty. The 'sex after SATs' approach is no longer considered adequate. This book and the other in this series (SRE 9–11) can be used to develop an SRE programme that spans several year groups — as a spiral curriculum.

What is SRE?

SRE (with both the biological and PSHE elements) is probably best defined in terms of what it aims to do. SRE/PSHE aims to help children and young people to develop:

★ self-esteem and self-awareness;

★ the skills needed for successful relationships;

★ a positive attitude towards difference and diversity;

★ an understanding of their own and others' rights;

★ emotional literacy;

★ the ability and confidence to make informed choices;

★ the knowledge, skills, understanding and attitude to optimise their health;

★ the ability and knowledge to keep themselves and other people safe by minimising risk from harm;

★ an understanding of their own and others' values and beliefs, and an individual moral framework that will help them to make well-considered decisions;

★ a discerning eye for the messages they receive from the media;

★ a positive attitude towards their body and sexuality;

★ the ability to access help and support.

From such aims, it is clear to see that SRE can be strongly linked to school ethos and is rarely delivered solely in discrete lessons. SRE can be frequently found in school assemblies, in the Social and Emotional Aspects of Learning (SEAL) curriculum, PSHE and the many conversations between adults and children that happen in school.

Why is SRE so important?

We teach our children to cross the road safely when they are very young because to do it dangerously could end up in injury or death. The consequences of decisions to do with sex, self-image and relationships can have a significant impact on a young person's life. SRE aims to help children and young people to make informed choices. If a child or young person has received effective SRE, it could ultimately impact positively upon:

★ the age at which a person first has sex;

★ the likelihood of a person contracting a sexually transmitted infection (STI);

★ the likelihood of an unplanned pregnancy (and/or teenage conception);

★ the likelihood of entering into an exploitative relationship;

★ emotional health and well-being;

★ the chance of developing a positive body image and self-esteem;

★ the likelihood of a young person accessing help and support with matters relating to the body or sex.

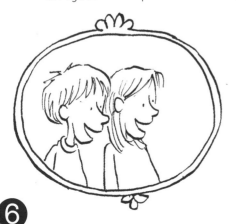

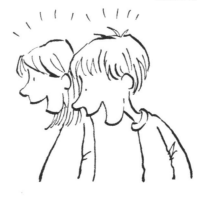

Why do we need SRE in Key Stage 2?

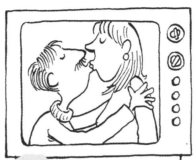

What children learn anyway

Children receive images of suggested sex at a very early age from a variety of sources (e.g. television, shop posters, magazines, graffiti, peers etc.). The messages children accept from these sources are often unrealistic, inaccurate and/or can cause prejudice. In addition, children can also pick up the message that talking about sex-related topics is forbidden. This can often mean that children have nobody reliable with which to discuss the information they receive and are often left feeling confused. A sensitively taught SRE programme at Key Stage 2 acts as a catch-all for those pupils whose parents/carers are uncomfortable talking about sex-related topics and will hopefully challenge the unhealthy and inaccurate messages many children receive.

It's not just about sex

Sex and Relationship Education is not just about the biology. Effective SRE does not focus on the facts alone. It needs to give pupils the opportunity to develop skills such as assertiveness, effective communication, responsible decision making and self-awareness, as well as providing the opportunity to explore and develop their own values and opinions (which will subsequently help to contribute to each pupil developing their own individual moral framework).

The need to prevent undesirable outcomes

Children who feel good about themselves and are knowledgeable and confident about their own bodies are more likely to take care with their sexual behaviour and to have fulfilling relationships when they enter into them later in life. If a child has always received the message that talking about body parts is in some way 'rude' or 'naughty', when they are older they are unlikely to feel that they can turn to the adults in their lives for information, help and support to do with sexual matters. The taboo around these issues can leave young people feeling isolated and unsure of where to seek advice and support. This, in turn, can have a significant impact on the decisions young people do or don't make about sex.

Ignorance is not the same as innocence

Some very young children ask questions about sex and body parts (e.g. what's the difference between girls and boys?). Parents/carers that have spoken openly about sexual matters to their children from an early age would argue that their children are no less innocent than those who have not received the information. Children receive the information at their own level and make sense of it in their own way. Their innocence is not destroyed by receiving this information if spoken about sensitively. Research also clearly shows that effective SRE does not encourage children to experiment with sex. Furthermore, SRE can help children to learn to protect themselves.

Biology: what, when and why?

It is down to each individual school to agree upon the content of its SRE programme. However, in a Key Stage 2 SRE programme, you often find:

★ life cycles, growing up and development – from baby to adult (usually built upon what was learnt in Key Stage 1);

★ the right we have over our own bodies (usually revised from Key Stage 1);

★ the emotional and physical changes of puberty – often covered from Years 3 or 4 onwards because children are entering into puberty earlier than several decades ago. Even if there are children in Year 4 who are not themselves experiencing puberty, they need to be aware of, and sensitive to, their peers' experiences;

★ information about sex and reproduction – sexual intercourse, conception, pregnancy and birth – often covered from Years 4 or 5 onwards because children have usually received information about these topics from a variety of sources by this age – some not always very accurate or 'healthy';

★ body parts – naming sexual organs – alongside the puberty and reproduction lessons.

Barriers to effective SRE

The quality and quantity of SRE can vary considerably from school to school. Some schools prioritise the delivery of SRE whilst others avoid it altogether! This is true of both primary and secondary schools. There are several possible barriers that can prevent a school from adopting an effective SRE programme.

❶ The amount of SRE happening in schools – perception and reality

Unfortunately, a common misconception amongst the general public and media is that effective SRE has been happening in all schools for many years now. This can feed the idea that SRE has led to the current high rates of teenage pregnancy and sexually transmitted infections, for example, and imply SRE is therefore not a good thing. The reality is that there are some pockets of excellent practice in SRE but just as many, if not more, that fall a long way short of this.

❷ Not being given priority

In a timetable that is already extremely full, and with so many curriculum areas to cover, it is easy to see how PSHE and SRE can sometimes fail to be prioritised. However, schools that do consider PSHE to be a vital part of the curriculum often see the benefits, not only because of the increase in positive interactions and relationships in the school, but also because of the improved academic standards achieved by the pupils.

❸ A general misunderstanding

Because few adults are given time to consider the issue of SRE, people often revert to a 'gut reaction' towards the subject that probably comes from their own experiences of learning about sex and body matters from the adults in their childhood. There is still a tendency to consider that SRE 'corrupts' children and young people, and encourages them to experiment with sex. A well-considered SRE programme would certainly do neither.

❹ Lack of staff training

This can be a result of a school not prioritising SRE and/or a lack of available local training. If staff have not been given time to consider good practice in SRE, they can become anxious about 'saying the wrong thing' or becoming embarrassed. If a clear policy has not been developed with the involvement of all staff, some teachers can feel like they are working in isolation and making up their own rules as they go along. This can cause reluctance in staff to teach SRE. The materials in this book can be used to support INSET on SRE if none is available from your local authority.

❺ Fear of parents'/carers' responses to SRE

Significantly, less than 1% of parents/carers in the UK exercise their right to withdraw their children from SRE lessons. The vast majority of parents/carers are supportive of schools delivering SRE, especially if they have been involved in any development or review of the school's programme and policy.

Parents/carers tend to sit anywhere on this spectrum:

Completely comfortable with SRE	Extremely uncomfortable with SRE

Both ends can be equally supportive of a school's SRE programme – one end because it believes SRE is important, and the other because parents/carers are happy that they themselves are not having to have the chat with their children about 'the facts of life'.

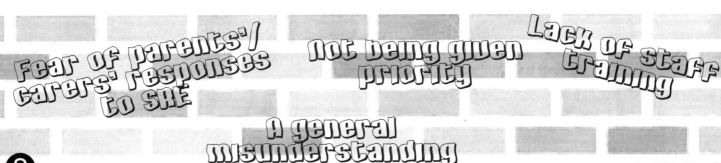

What is statutory in SRE?

Policy

It is a legal requirement that every school has an SRE policy. Currently in primary schools, this policy can state that no other sex and relationship education outside the relevant requirements of the National Curriculum Science Orders will take place. Few schools opt to have this as their policy. With the possibility of PSHE becoming statutory in the near future, this could all change. The headteacher and governors have ultimate responsibility for the SRE policy. It needs to be kept up-to-date and free copies made available to parents/carers on request.

Programme

The headteacher and governors also have the ultimate responsibility for approving the content of an SRE programme and its organisation, i.e. integrated or discrete, delivered, for example, through PSHE and/or Science. They should be satisfied that teaching materials are appropriate and that any contribution by outside speakers/agencies are consistent with the policy. Secondary schools are required to provide an SRE programme that includes, as a minimum, information about sexually transmitted infections and HIV/AIDS.

Parents'/carers' right to withdraw

Parents and carers have the right to withdraw their children from all or part of SRE provided at school, except for those parts included in the statutory National Curriculum. This right needs to be clearly stated in the school's SRE policy. The Statutory National Curriculum Science Order legally binds schools to teach the following elements of SRE in Key Stages 1 and 2:

Key Stage 1 (5−7 year olds)
Pupils should be taught:

★ that animals, including humans, move, feed, grow, use their senses and reproduce.

★ to recognise and compare the main external parts of the bodies of humans.

★ that humans and animals can produce offspring and that these grow into adults.

★ to recognise similarities and differences between themselves and others, and to treat others with sensitivity.

Key Stage 2 (7−11 year olds)
Pupils should be taught:

★ that the life processes common to humans and other animals include nutrition, growth and reproduction.

★ about the main stages of the human life cycle.

GOVERNMENT GUIDANCE
(non-statutory)

The most recent (non-statutory) government guidance produced for SRE is the document:
Sex and Relationship Education Guidance 0116/200.
Downloadable from:
http://www.dfes.gov.uk/sreguidance/sexeducation.pdf

What's in a Name?

★ PSHE and citizenship— Personal, Social and Health Education and citizenship. All of the currently non-statutory PSHE curriculum. Found at: http://www.teachernet.gov.uk/ZPSHE/curriculum.cfm?sectionId=76

★ SRE – Sex and Relationship Education —a large part of PSHE. Sex education became SRE in the year 2000 in an attempt to prevent a sole focus on biology.

★ Sex Education – the 'sex bits' of SRE.

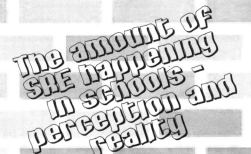

The amount of SRE happening in schools - perception and reality

A guide to good practice in SRE

This section provides a summary of what is currently deemed good practice in SRE and includes tips that can help to make the experience of delivering it more comfortable.

Ground rules

Ground rules can significantly impact on the comfort of both the teacher and pupils during an SRE lesson. They are best developed in consensus with everyone in the room. Many of the ground rules the children suggest might be similar to the class rules you developed at the start of the year. However, in SRE lessons it is usually wise to ensure there is a rule that:

★ makes sure that no personal questions are asked. (This does not mean people cannot volunteer personal information.);

★ acknowledges possible embarrassment and provides a strategy to deal with it (e.g. an opt-out moment). You might also like to include a rule that encourages everyone to be respectful about other pupils' and your (the teacher's) possible embarrassment;

★ states that no one should laugh at anyone else's contribution to these lessons;

★ helps you (the teacher) to deal comfortably with any questions that arise (see the section 'Dealing with questions');

★ makes it clear that if you deem anyone to be at risk from harm, you will have to go to tell another adult.

Use the correct terms for body parts

It is a good idea to use the correct terms for body parts in SRE lessons. The reasons for this are:

★ It equips pupils with the correct terms that they will hopefully feel comfortable using in future, for example, with health professionals.

★ A lot of slang is derogatory.

★ You could never accommodate every pupil's family name for sexual organs – although there is no harm in acknowledging them.

★ It will create consistency throughout the school and in every SRE lesson.

Dealing with questions

Undoubtedly, the issue that can cause teachers the most anxiety in SRE lessons are the sexually explicit questions that pupils may ask out of the blue. There are two basic approaches to answering questions that a school might adopt as policy:

❶ Answer every question any pupil asks – there on the spot.

❷ Provide a question box and explain that you will answer questions that are to do with the topic in hand but any other questions need to be placed in the box and answered at a later time. Furthermore, you can also use this box as a 'buffer' for any question a pupil asks that you do not want to answer on the spot by saying: *'I would like to think about that question before I answer it. Do you mind writing it down and putting it in the question box?'* This gives you time to consult with other members of staff if you feel you need to and also to consider your answer!

By using the second method, you can remove the anxiety of the unexpected. You could mention this deferred answering as a ground rule that you (the teacher) would like to have included.

Extreme embarrassment

If a member of staff is extremely uneasy about topics taught in SRE, they are unlikely to do a good job and could possibly give pupils unhealthy messages about sex and body parts. A school might adopt a 'get out' clause in their SRE policy for such teachers and allow another teacher (known to the pupils) to deliver it. It might also be a good idea for this member of staff to be offered SRE training.

Giggling

Teachers sometimes complain about pupils laughing during SRE lessons and 'not taking the lessons seriously'. However, on further reflection, it is easy to see that the giggling is a result of the pupils' awkwardness with the subject. It is easy to forget that pupils will have picked up on the taboo nature of SRE issues. The following could help with this issue:

❶ Start the lesson deliberately setting out for a good giggle e.g. play a game where some pupils have to shout out the definitions of words from SRE lessons and other pupils shout out the actual word. This also helps pupils to learn the correct terms and their meanings.

❷ Don't be afraid of giggling yourself. Explain you were caught a little off-guard!

★ Brainstorm some questions (or use those in the question box if you have one) and practise the answers.

★ If you are comfortable with talking about the idea of sex in terms of pleasure — not just in terms of reproduction — it helps to overcome some embarrassment.

★ If you believe a pupil is shouting out a question just to cause embarrassment, you could try asking him or her what they think the answer is or, better still, just answer frankly!

★ You will probably feel safer sticking to frank, factual answers. Have these prepared!

★ Remember that you never have to answer personal questions. Not asking personal questions should be part of the ground rules — make this very clear at the beginning of each SRE lesson. Make sure the ground rules are displayed and refer to them if reminders are needed.

★ Many sexual acts can be described in terms of touching different parts of the body because it feels nice, without going into very explicit detail.

❸ Start the first session by openly discussing why people feel awkward talking about sex. You could discuss the legacy of the Victorian era and how a taboo can have detrimental effects on decisions that teenagers and adults make about sexual health.

Most teachers find that after some initial giggling, pupils soon settle down and become interested in the topic.

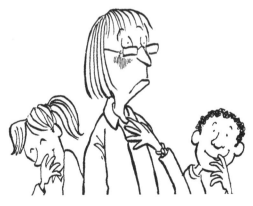

Mixed- or single-sex groups

It is generally deemed good practice that both sexes learn about each other. In many schools, both male and female pupils have the majority of their SRE lessons in mixed-sex groups, but are then given a session where boys are grouped with a male teacher and girls with a female teacher. In these single-sex groups, both sexes will feel more comfortable asking questions. Some schools teach all SRE lessons in single-sex groups.

Differentiation

Sometimes, because of the subject matter, SRE is taught in a way (using cross-section diagrams for example) that can leave less able pupils confused. If these pupils receive extra support outside the classroom, it is a good idea for them to have the opportunity to talk through what they have learnt in SRE lessons in a smaller group with more support to check that there have been no major misunderstandings (e.g. that boys have periods).

Inclusivity

SRE needs to be inclusive. To effectively do this, it needs to acknowledge (or even celebrate) the full spectrum of diversity found in humankind and avoid making assumptions, generalisations or stereotypes about people's sexuality, race, religion, family set-ups, culture, social background etc. Efforts need to be made not to promote any one group as 'the norm' and SRE resources will ideally portray the diversity found in society. Furthermore, prejudice should always be challenged.

Active learning

Just sitting pupils in front of a video/DVD with no opportunity to ask questions has limited impact. Effective SRE uses active learning techniques, which means that pupils get actively involved in their own learning. Active learning techniques can include any tool that prompts discussion and collaborative ideas development. Here are some examples:

★ Prioritising activities – sort anything from the most significant to the least significant, or choose the single most important issue and explain why it is important.

★ Carousels – ask pupils to sit in two concentric circles, with the inside circle facing outwards and the outside circle facing inwards. A topic is discussed for a few minutes between opposite pairs. After this, either the inner or outer circle moves one seat to the left or right, and the same topic is discussed and developed further with a new person.

★ Agreement spectra – explain to the pupils that an imaginary line is a spectrum. Down one end is 'strongly agree' and down the other is 'strongly disagree'. Read out a statement and ask pupils to stand on a spectrum in a place that best represents how they feel about what was said. Invite pupils to discuss the issue by asking, 'Who would like to say anything about where they are standing?'.

★ Puzzles and games – try mix and match, true or false or draw a fact and ask others to guess it.

★ Presentations – set pupils the challenge of making a leaflet, advert, presentation, skit, poster, collage etc. to present to the rest of the class.

★ Brainstorm using graffiti walls – ask pupils to write ideas on different sheets that relate to different topics.

★ Role play, hot seating and freeze frames – use drama methods to explore a dilemma, choice, crisis etc.

★ Interview questions – ask pupils to consider questions they would like to have answered on a particular issue by an expert.

★ Use picture prompts – to facilitate discussions about any particular issue.

Preaching or facilitating?

Everyone is entitled to their own personal views and to make choices that are based on their own values – as long as these views or values do not impact on the rights of others. As teachers, it is helpful to have a clear understanding of our own views so that we have an awareness of what we might be imparting unwittingly to our pupils. For example, as an individual, you might believe strongly that for you, eating meat is wrong. However, this might not be the view of some of the children and their parents/carers in your class and it would be inappropriate for you to push this view as the only 'correct' one. Effective SRE does not promote one viewpoint. It explores all viewpoints and the teacher is the facilitator for this exploration, not the person who promotes one view as 'correct'. Positive values common to all humankind can, however, be promoted. These might include respect for others, anti-prejudice, honesty, never deliberately harming others, etc., which are likely to echo your school rules and ethos.

The table below is a summary of two different approaches to teaching PSHE and SRE. Pro-choice teaching can be more effective in helping pupils to become equipped to make their own decisions. This table can best be explained by example. Restricted choice would be if a teacher said to a class, 'Never smoke – it is bad for you'. In comparison, a pro-choice teacher may say, 'When you grow up, you might decide never to smoke or you might decide to become a smoker. It will be a decision that you might have to make at some point. Let's explore the possible consequences of each choice'. Then you could explore the negative impact of smoking and the reasons why someone might start smoking.

Restricted-choice teaching...	Pro-choice teaching...
can consider one point of view to be the right one and imposes this on others.	respects that everyone is entitled to their own point of view as long as these views do not impact on the rights of others.
can be biased, judgemental and moralistic.	gets pupils to consider the issues relating to a personal choice or circumstance in a non-judgemental way.
does not give pupils the full picture and does not acknowledge the full spectrum of diversity and/or choice.	gives pupils the full picture and acknowledges the full spectrum of diversity.
tells pupils what is right and what is wrong.	encourages pupils to explore issues together with the aim of them understanding and developing their own individual moral framework.
is sometimes appropriate for teaching young children e.g. this is how you cross the road.	helps children to develop independence and an ability to make their own choices as they grow up.
tells pupils not to do certain things e.g. don't smoke.	explains everything in terms of choices e.g. 'you might be someone who will smoke when you are older, you might not . . . let's consider the choices and their impact'.
can involve scaremongering and making one choice seem awful.	looks at realistic risks and how to reduce them.
tries to 'protect' children and young people by withholding information from them.	aims to 'equip' children and young people.
sends the message 'We choose for you.'	sends the message 'You learn to choose for yourself.'

Evaluating, assessing and monitoring

As with other subjects, the following can help to maintain and improve the quality of this subject, and opportunities for this need to be included in any planning:

★ pupils' and teachers' evaluations of lessons and/or topics;
★ pupils' self-assessments/teachers' assessments;
★ the PSHE coordinator's monitoring of SRE.

A whole-school approach

As with any change in school, if the whole school community is invited to join in with the process, the outcome is far more likely to be adopted and sustained by everyone. Overnight changes implemented by one person usually have little impact. With SRE, getting people to 'buy in' to the idea is crucial and probably where 50% of the effort needs to go. Here are some suggestions for involving various groups of the school community in the review or development of your school's SRE.

Involving pupils

Pupils could be involved by:

★ asking the school council to view the resources and making suggestions about their use, or by carrying out other investigations such as:
  - Do boys and girls have different attitudes to SRE?
  - Just how embarrassing is SRE and what makes it embarrassing?
  - What makes a good SRE teacher?
  - What TV programmes are children in different year groups allowed to watch? (To see what sex and relationship issues and images pupils are already exposed to.)
★ asking Year 6 to produce a pupil-friendly version of the policy.
★ answering a questionnaire about SRE (an example can be found on page 63).

Involving parent/carers

Many children express a preference for their parents/carers teaching them about SRE matters. Unfortunately, not all parents/carers are comfortable with this and would prefer to leave it to the school. However, any support materials that can be sent home as leaflets or homework that is to be completed with a parent/carer can encourage a degree of their involvement.

Most schools inform and consult parents and carers about SRE. As a minimum, parents/carers need to be given information prior to the SRE lessons outlining what will be covered and reminding them of their right to withdraw their child from these sessions. An example of such a pre-programme letter can be found on page 59. Better practice is to also consult with parents/carers each time the school's SRE programme and policy are reviewed. This could be done using a consultation form such as that found on page 62.

Many schools also run evening or afternoon sessions for parents/carers to look at SRE. In any session you run for parents/carers, you need to be mindful of what you wish to achieve. Your aims might include:

❶ helping parents/carers to see that SRE is a positive thing;
❷ helping parents/carers to support the school's programme by continuing conversations at home;
❸ showing parents/carers an outline of the main topics that will be covered.

Information for parents/carers that aims to help them to understand and feel positive about SRE can be found on pages 60–61. This could be sent out with a consultation form or with a pre-programme letter. Some of the training activities in this book would be appropriate for use with parents/carers. It is also good practice to inform parents/carers of their right to a free copy of the school's SRE policy, although few take up this offer.

Staff

A staff meeting (or two) that covers the key issues of SRE is the best way to involve staff. Possible content might include:

★ What is SRE?
★ What does SRE aim to do?
★ SRE as part of the PSHE curriculum – it's not just about sex.
★ Exploring our own experiences and attitudes towards SRE.
★ Why do we need SRE at Key Stage 2?
★ What is good practice in SRE and what will help us to feel more comfortable delivering it?
★ The school's SRE programme.
★ The school's SRE policy.

Such a staff meeting could be delivered using the materials in this book, although some local authorities do provide SRE training.

Governors

Many schools have a governor with responsibility for PSHE and SRE. It might be appropriate for this governor to attend an SRE staff meeting, as well as discussing information about SRE specifically in a governors' meeting.

Training activities

The next few pages contain training activities that can be used with school staff, parents/carers and governors. Most activities are based on a photocopiable sheet.

Rosie and Jack
– uses the photocopiable sheet on page 17.

Purpose of activity: to show that effective SRE is about more than children and young people just knowing facts.

Suitable audiences: school staff, parents/carers and governors.

Method of delivery: read through the scenario. Ask what the potential negative outcomes of this situation are (e.g. unplanned pregnancy, sexually transmitted infection (STI), regret, nasty rumours, loss of self-respect etc.). See if everyone agrees that it is not an ideal situation, then ask pairs or groups of three to discuss where each of the skills at the bottom of the sheet could have 'kicked in' to prevent the outcome.

Key discussion points:
- ★ SRE is not just about facts. It is also about skills and values.
- ★ Young people need to learn the facts about sex, but considering real-life situations and learning skills, such as assertiveness, are more likely to positively impact on the decisions young people make than the facts alone.
- ★ SRE is embedded in the PSHE curriculum.

Considering the SRE we received when we were at school

Purpose of activity: to reflect upon our own school's SRE and the messages it gave us.

Suitable audiences: school staff, parents/carers and governors.

Method of delivery: ask pairs or groups of three to consider each of the following questions:

❶ What do you remember being taught in your school's SRE?

❷ Was your school's SRE just dominated by biology, or were there discussions about relationships?

❸ What are your memories of your teachers' approach to SRE?

❹ What would have made the SRE you received more useful?

Key discussion points:
- ★ Many people's experience of their school's SRE is less than brilliant. It usually only focused on biology, often only referred to rabbits or frogs, and there were rarely opportunities to ask questions.
- ★ People often recall lessons that left them confused or worried. If delivered well, SRE does not leave children confused.
- ★ The quality and quantity of SRE in different schools still varies considerably.
- ★ SRE needs to be 'normalised' so that children get the impression that adults can talk about sex and the body.

Considering our own attitudes and values towards SRE

Purpose of activity: to consider different responses to, and levels of comfort with, SRE.

Suitable audiences: school staff, parents/carers and governors.

Method of delivery: ask pairs or groups of three to consider each of these questions:

❶ At what age do you think children should first learn about the following in this school's SRE:
- ★ the changes of puberty;
- ★ sexual intercourse?

Allow people to volunteer their thoughts. Discuss their

suggestions and interject the key points below. Then ask everyone to discuss in pairs the following question:

❷ What do you think people's fears are about SRE? Discuss the answers as a whole group.

Key discussion points:

★ Everyone will have different ideas for suitable ages.

★ Considering that children start puberty as young as eight now, the changes of puberty are probably best covered from about Years 3 or 4 onwards – in a sensitive and simple way.

★ Children are exposed to so many images of suggested sex from a variety of sources (the media, peers, older siblings, graffiti etc.). The information children receive from these sources is not always healthy or accurate. It could be argued that it is better that children receive this information from a sensitively taught, accurate SRE programme.

★ It is down to each individual school to agree on the content of an SRE programme and when it is taught.

★ The fears that people usually have about SRE usually come from their own poor experiences of SRE.

What messages do we want children and young people to receive?

– uses the photocopiable sheet on page 18.

Purpose of activity: to consider the messages we do and don't want children and young people to receive from their SRE.

Suitable audiences: school staff.

Method of delivery: ask pairs to sort through each message and decide whether they think it is a suitable message or not for children and young people.

Key discussion points:

★ It is a good idea to consider the underlying messages you might want children to receive about sex and body parts. Sometimes we give negative messages inadvertently.

★ Messages we might want to promote include: sex can be a positive thing (it doesn't just give you STIs and unplanned pregnancies), you can talk to trusted adults about any worries you have about puberty and sex, some people do feel uncomfortable talking about sex and sometimes they show

Concerns of teachers	What addresses the fear?
Parents/carers will complain about the content.	Most parents/carers are supportive of the SRE a school delivers, especially if they have been consulted about it. The minority that do not agree with the programme can exercise their right to withdraw their child from these sessions.
I might say the wrong thing.	Guidance given earlier in this section about answering questions shows how you can engineer some time to consider your answers

Concerns of parents/carers	What addresses the fear?
The information will scare the children.	If it is taught well, it should not scare the children.
Teachers don't know what they are doing.	Teachers will receive training and resources.
This information will encourage children to experiment.	Research has shown that effective SRE does not do this. The average age of first sex in the Netherlands, where a far more consistent and comprehensive approach to SRE is adopted, is higher than in the UK.
Views different from my own might be taught.	SRE is never about promoting one viewpoint. A person's right to a different viewpoint (that does not impact on the rights of others) is respected.
My child will come home and ask me questions.	Parents/carers can be supported with this by sending resources home with the child. Parent/carers will be informed about the programme prior to delivery.

this by giggling (which is fine), we celebrate difference and diversity, sexual stereotyping is not helpful, you have the right to access help and support, you have the right not to be touched if you do not want to, there is behaviour that is unacceptable in public etc.

★ The 'abortion is wrong' card highlights that whatever our personal view is, it is not our place to promote it in the classroom.

★ The 'boys have periods' card highlights that plenty of opportunities for pupils to ask questions and differentiation are part of effective SRE.

Equip or protect?
– uses the photocopiable sheet on page 19.

Purpose of activity: to understand that as children grow up, they need to be equipped to deal with life circumstances because they cannot forever be protected by the adults in their lives.

Suitable audiences: school staff, parents/carers and governors.

Method of delivery: define and compare the terms 'equip' and 'protect' as follows:

Equip: to give children the skills and information that mean they can protect themselves.

Protect: to keep children away from anything that is a real or perceived source of potential harm.

Look at each scenario and decide whether each is equipping or protecting a child.

Key discussion points:

★ It is completely appropriate for very young children to be 'protected' as they have not yet developed the skills or gained the knowledge to protect themselves (e.g. a two year old would put their finger in a plug socket if left unattended).

★ As children grow up and become more independent, we cannot realistically expect to follow them around for every single minute of every day. Because of this, we do need to start to equip them for any potential situations or hazards that they might encounter. For example, we teach children to cross the road by themselves when we are sure they can do so safely.

★ Some parents/carers want to protect their children from information about sex because they believe the information will be dangerous. Other parents/carers take the view that their children will eventually discover sex anyway and therefore it is better to start talking about these issues before their child encounters them. Furthermore, these parents'/carers' open attitude might mean that their child would more willingly turn to them for advice and support about matters to do with sex.

Media images

Purpose of activity: to consider the unhealthy messages children and young people receive from the media and other sources, and to help everyone to see that a SRE programme is a better source of information.

Suitable audiences: school staff, parents/carers and governors.

Method of delivery: collect a variety of media images. Images from a magazine aimed at young adults will suffice but if you have time, use a camera to collect examples of graffiti, shop displays/posters and cartoons. Also try to collect images or quotes from internet sites or computer games, pop video images, TV programmes and quotations from pupils that show misunderstandings or prejudices, quotations from parents/carers unwilling to talk about sex etc. Scatter these images around the room for people to look at. Ask, 'What messages do our children receive about sex, gender and relationships from these sources?'. At the end, discuss this question as a group.

Key discussion points:

Children and young people can be bombarded with these images. Some of the untrue and unhealthy messages they receive include:

★ Everyone is having sex all the time.

★ Sex is exciting, fun, easy and uncomplicated.

★ There are very narrow ideas about what is attractive.

★ Straight relationships are the only 'normal' ones.

★ Your worth is based on what you look like.

★ It's not cool to be academic.

★ Sex is too embarrassing to talk about with adults.

One of the aims of SRE is to challenge these messages.

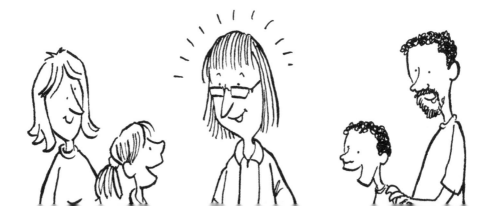

Rosie and Jack

Rosie and Jack are both 16. Rosie has just finished with her boyfriend with whom she had a sexual relationship. She is quite angry and upset about this. Jack has never had a girlfriend.

Rosie and Jack are at a party. They are both drinking alcohol and feel pretty drunk. Jack has always fancied Rosie but he has never had the courage to start up a conversation with her. He keeps looking at Rosie but she doesn't seem to be noticing him. Jack's mate Ben teases him about Rosie and says he should stop messing about and go and 'get in there'.

Jack walks over to Rosie. The music is really loud so they can't really hear what each other is trying to say. Rosie leads Jack out of the room, up the stairs and into a bedroom. She kisses Jack. She wants Jack to like her. They then proceed to have unprotected sex that neither of them particularly enjoy.

Consider each of the following. Where could they each have 'kicked in' to prevent what happened and what might have changed?

1. knowing how to keep yourself safe and reduce risk
2. resisting peer pressure
3. challenging media messages
4. the ability to access help and support
5. being able to communicate openly
6. awareness of real-life dilemmas
7. being responsible
8. planning ahead
9. being able to express how you feel
10. self-esteem
11. making informed decisions
12. understanding the impact that alcohol has on your judgement
13. respect for others
14. negotiation skills
15. knowing about different types of relationships
16. empathy
17. self-awareness
18. factual knowledge about alcohol
19. factual knowledge about sex

What 'messages' do we want children and young people to receive from their SRE?

Sex is something adults never talk about.	There are parts of the body that are disgusting.
You should never be pressurised into doing something you do not want to do.	You should never pick on another person for any real or perceived difference.
Boys have to behave differently from girls.	If you giggle about sex you are childish.
If you cannot sort out a problem yourself, you need to find help.	There are parts of the body that you should not touch, in a place where other people can see you.
If anyone touches you in a way you do not like, you have the right to stop it from happening.	Sex is disgusting.
Life has risks but there are usually things you can do to make yourself as safe as possible.	Being straight is the only 'normal' type of relationship.
Sex is just a biological function.	Sex is something adults do and it is usually best in a loving, trusting and caring relationship.
The decision to have a sexual relationship with someone needs some thought.	Sex always gives you STIs and unplanned pregnancies.
Abortion is wrong.	Boys have periods.

Equip or protect?

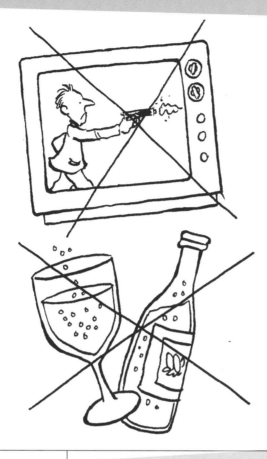

When you teach your five year old how to cross the road safely.	When you don't let your 14 year old see a leaflet about safer sex in the doctor's waiting room.	When you put your two year old in a play pen whilst you answer the phone.
When you discuss the changes of puberty with your eight year old.	When you stop your five year old from seeing violence on the television.	When you don't let your 15 year old go to any parties.
When you tell your nine year old you have never smoked when you have.	When you tell your 11 year old about how friends can sometimes put pressure on each other to do things they might not want to do.	When you teach your four year old not to put their finger in a plug socket.
When you give your 16 year old a pack of condoms and talk with them about safer sex and how they might know if they are ready for a sexual relationship.	When you discuss with your 12 year old how alcohol makes you feel.	When you tell your 15 year old never to drink alcohol.

What would we expect to find in a Key Stage 2 SRE programme?

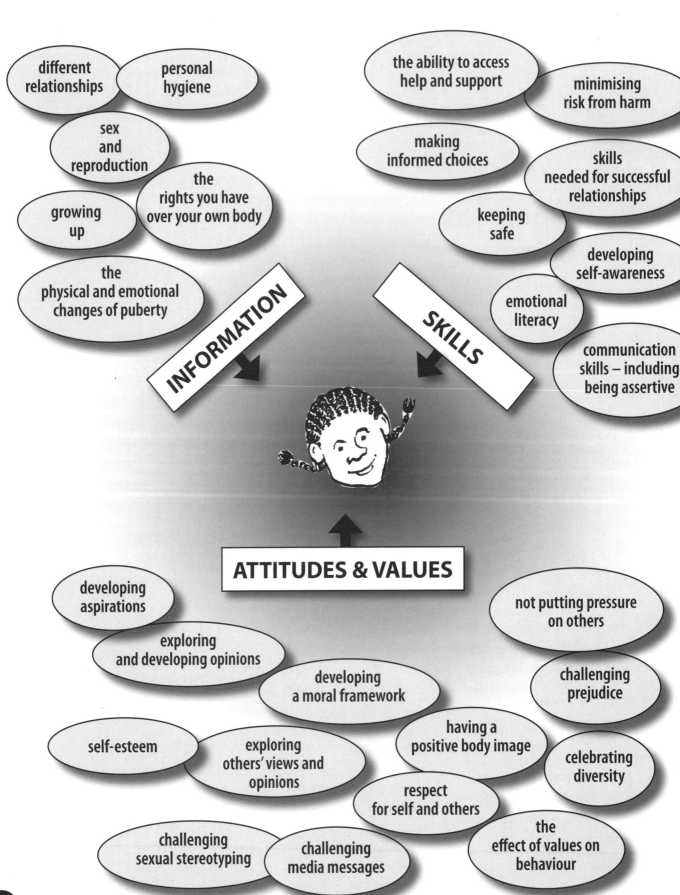

different relationships

personal hygiene

sex and reproduction

the rights you have over your own body

growing up

the physical and emotional changes of puberty

the ability to access help and support

minimising risk from harm

making informed choices

skills needed for successful relationships

keeping safe

developing self-awareness

emotional literacy

communication skills – including being assertive

INFORMATION

SKILLS

ATTITUDES & VALUES

developing aspirations

exploring and developing opinions

developing a moral framework

self-esteem

exploring others' views and opinions

having a positive body image

respect for self and others

challenging sexual stereotyping

challenging media messages

the effect of values on behaviour

not putting pressure on others

challenging prejudice

celebrating diversity

SRE policy

POLICY DEVELOPMENT

As with most documentation, the value of an SRE policy is in the discussions and considerations its development prompts. Involving the whole school community (pupils, school staff, parents/carers and governors) in the production of an SRE policy is considered best practice.

an SRE policy Needs to:

★ define SRE;
★ describe the consultation process that took place during the policy development;
★ outline the content of the school's SRE programme;
★ provide a secure framework for staff to work within;
★ include a statement of the underlying values on which the SRE programme is based;
★ give details of SRE provision, for example, timetabling and who delivers it;
★ give details of the member of staff responsible for SRE development and coordination;
★ describe how SRE will be monitored and evaluated;
★ state that parents have the legal right to withdraw their child from SRE;
★ give an outline of the provision for regular review of the policy.

an SRE policy could be documented using the following headings:

a. Introduction
b. Background Information
c. Policy Statement
d. Aims and Objectives
  – of the policy
  – of the SRE programme
e. Moral and Values Framework
f. Equal Opportunities Statement
g. Content
h. Organisation
i. Specific Issues within SRE
j. Dissemination of the Policy

Policy development guidance

The following framework provides suggestions and examples that could be included in each of the sections (listed on the previous page) of an SRE policy.

a. INTRODUCTION

Name of school
Date of policy
Member(s) of staff responsible
Review date

b. BACKGROUND INFORMATION

★ A description of the school, including the geography and setting, local health and social priorities, number of pupils on roll, ethnic and religious mix, and special needs of pupils.

★ A description of the policy development, including the consultation process with pupils, parents/carers, governors, external agencies and the community.

c. THE POLICY STATEMENT

What is Sex and Relationship Education (SRE)?
Possible definitions

SRE is embedded in the PSHE curriculum and aims to help children to develop:

★ self-esteem and self-awareness;
★ the skills needed for successful relationships;
★ a positive attitude towards difference and diversity;
★ an understanding of their own and others' rights;
★ emotional literacy;
★ the ability and confidence to make informed choices;
★ the knowledge, skills, understanding and attitude to optimise their health;
★ the ability and knowledge to keep themselves and other people safe by minimising risk from harm;
★ an understanding of their own and others' values and beliefs, and an individual moral framework that will help them to make well-considered decisions;
★ a discerning eye for the messages they receive from the media;
★ a positive attitude towards their body and sexuality;
★ the ability to access help and support.

SRE gives pupils accurate information about sex and relationships, and allows them the opportunities to develop life skills and an individual moral framework that aims to enable them to make positive use of that information.

Why should SRE be taught?
Possible reasons

★ In a world where children receive information about sex and relationships from a variety of sources, many of which are inaccurate or 'unhealthy', primary school SRE aims to counterbalance these messages by providing accurate information as part of a supportive programme.

★ SRE is about helping children to develop and maintain successful relationships. It is about providing them with information that will support them with the process of puberty and help them to understand issues relating to sex and reproduction.

★ Primary school SRE needs to happen at a time when many children start to experience puberty and show an increased awareness of matters relating to the body and sex.

★ Primary school SRE is about demonstrating to children that matters relating to the body and sex can be spoken about in a sensitive and positive way. This helps children to feel more comfortable about communicating about these matters. This therefore will undoubtedly increase the likelihood of them behaving responsibly in any sexual relationship they go on to have, as such responsibility usually requires some kind of communication – with a partner and/or sexual health services.

Legal requirements

The law in relation to SRE states:

'The governing bodies of schools are required to keep an up-to-date SRE policy that describes the content and organisation of SRE provided outside the National Curriculum Science Orders.'

'Parents/carers have the right to withdraw their children from SRE lessons.'

Other related policies and documents

The SRE policy can also be linked to other policies:

Confidentiality Policy
PSHE Policy
Safeguarding Children Policy
Drug Education Policy
Teaching and Learning Policy
Inclusion Policy

d. AIMS AND OBJECTIVES

The policy
What are the aims and objectives of the policy?

For example:
This policy is a working document which provides guidance and information on all aspects of SRE, and aims to provide a secure framework within which staff can work.

Audience

Those who should read the policy are:
★ staff

- ★ parents/carers
- ★ governors
- ★ visitors to the school.

This policy is referred to in the school's prospectus where parents and carers are also informed of their right to withdraw their child from SRE lessons. A free copy of the SRE policy is available on request from the school.

The SRE programme
Possible statements

Our SRE programme aims to provide children with:
- ★ the skills needed for successful relationships;
- ★ a moral framework that will guide their decisions and behaviours;
- ★ opportunities to understand and celebrate difference and diversity;
- ★ an understanding of their own bodies;
- ★ the confidence and know-how to seek help and advice;
- ★ self-esteem, self-awareness and emotional health;
- ★ an awareness of the right they have over their own body;
- ★ good communication skills – including assertiveness;
- ★ the skills and knowledge to make positive informed choices;
- ★ the ability to respect the rights of others to hold opinions that differ from their own as long as these views do not impact on the rights of anyone else;
- ★ the ability to take responsibility for, and accept the consequences of, their own actions;
- ★ the knowledge to reduce the risks to their own health and the health of others.

e. MORAL AND VALUES FRAMEWORK

What values does our primary school wish to promote as a moral framework within which to teach SRE?
Possible statements

Our primary school teaches SRE within the following moral and values framework, which promotes:
- ★ self-respect and respect for others;
- ★ empathy, mutual support and cooperation;
- ★ honesty;
- ★ responsibility for personal actions;
- ★ an awareness of the uniqueness of individuals;
- ★ respect and acceptance towards others who may have different backgrounds, cultures and sexuality;
- ★ an awareness of not making assumptions about others;
- ★ the right of people to hold their own views (as long as these views do not impact negatively on the rights of others);
- ★ the right not to be abused or taken advantage of by other people;
- ★ the right to accurate information about sex and relationship issues.

f. EQUAL OPPORTUNITIES STATEMENT

Statement of our school's commitment to equal opportunities and inclusion, with reference to our school's Inclusion and Equal Opportunities Policies
Possible statements

Our primary school is committed to the provision of SRE to all of its pupils. Equal time and provision will be allocated to all pupils with the exception of pupils with special educational needs, who will be given extra support.

Our SRE programme is inclusive and acknowledges and accommodates the diversity within any group of people in terms of gender, religion, language, race, social background, culture, appearance, family set-up, special needs, ability or disability.

g. CONTENT

Outline of our primary school's SRE programme, including what is covered in each year group/Key Stage.

Every school needs to develop its own SRE programme. There needs to be agreement about which topics will be covered in which year groups (and which will be revisited in more than one year group e.g. puberty). The content of SRE (embedded in PSHE) at Key Stage 2 might include several of the following topics:
- ★ the physical and emotional changes of puberty
- ★ sex and reproduction
- ★ growing up
- ★ naming sexual organs
- ★ personal hygiene
- ★ challenging sexual stereotyping
- ★ challenging homophobia
- ★ considering media messages
- ★ developing a positive body image
- ★ changing relationships as we grow up
- ★ aspirations and how we might see our futures
- ★ different types of relationship
- ★ how to find help and support
- ★ developing emotional literacy
- ★ peer influence and peer pressure
- ★ considering rights and responsibilities
- ★ raising self-esteem and increasing self-awareness
- ★ exploring friendships – making, valuing and maintaining them
- ★ challenging assumptions, stereotyping and prejudice
- ★ communication skills – saying 'no', being assertive and dealing with conflict, negotiation and appreciation.

How was the content decided?
Possible statements

- ★ A needs assessment was carried out.
- ★ Pupils' prior knowledge was investigated.
- ★ The SRE policy development working party met to consider content.
- ★ Consultation with staff, pupils, parents/carers, governors and external agencies took place.
- ★ Local and national guidance was considered.

How are resources used? (with reasons for their selection)
For example

SRE resources are chosen and checked for:
- ★ inclusivity
- ★ positive, healthy and unbiased messages
- ★ age appropriateness
- ★ promoting positive values
- ★ accuracy
- ★ being up-to-date.

h. ORGANISATION

How is SRE delivered?
For example

SRE is:
* embedded in the PSHE curriculum;
* delivered in PSHE lessons for each year group in the first half of the summer term;
* delivered in both Science and PSHE lessons.

Who delivers SRE?
An example statement

SRE is delivered predominantly by the pupils' class teacher. In Year 6, the school nurse enhances the programme by delivering two informal sessions on the changes of puberty.

How does our school use outside agencies?
An example statement

Occasionally, appropriate and suitably-experienced and/or knowledgeable visitors from outside the school may be invited to contribute to the delivery of SRE in our school. Our school has a code of practice for using visitors to support the delivery of PSHE:
* Visitors are invited into school because of the particular expertise or contribution they are able to make.
* All visitors are familiar with and understand the school's SRE policy and work within it.
* All input into PSHE lessons is part of a planned programme and negotiated and agreed with staff in advance.
* All visitors are supervised/supported by a member of staff at all times.
* The input of visitors is monitored and evaluated by staff and pupils. This evaluation informs future planning.

How will the SRE programme be monitored and evaluated?
For example

* Questionnaires
* Discussions
* Teacher assessments
* Pupils' self-assessment and evaluations
* Teacher evaluations at the end of a block of lessons, which are then forwarded to the PSHE coordinator to inform future developments.

How does our school keep parents/carers informed of the SRE programme?
For example

Before any year group embarks upon its SRE programme, parents/carers are informed by letter of their right to withdraw their child from SRE lessons. They are given an overview of the topics the child will be covering. Parents/carers are also reminded that they can have a copy of the school's SRE policy on request.

i. SPECIFIC ISSUES WITHIN SRE

What provision does our school make for those pupils withdrawn from SRE lessons?
For example

Parents/carers have the right to withdraw their child from all or part of the sex and relationship education provided at school except for those parts included in statutory National Curriculum. Those parents/carers wishing to exercise this right are invited to discuss their objections and concerns, and to reflect on the impact withdrawal may have on the child. Once a child has been withdrawn, they cannot take part in the SRE programme until the request for withdrawal has been removed. Materials are available to parents/carers who wish to supplement the school SRE programme or who wish to deliver SRE to their children at home.

Safeguarding children statement
For example

SRE may bring about disclosures of safeguarding children issues and all staff are familiar with the procedures for reporting their concerns. In these cases, the school's safeguarding children policy needs to be referred to.

Confidentiality Statement
Possible statements

As a general rule, a child's confidentiality is maintained by the teacher or member of staff concerned. However, if this person believes that the child is at risk or in danger, they talk to the named child protection coordinator who may or may not confer with the head teacher before any decision is made. (This is generally considered good practice.)

Our school will offer absolutely no confidentiality – and make it clear to both pupils and parents that this is the case. For example, we would pass on information about a parent/carer breaking the law if it were disclosed to us – even if the child was at no risk from harm. (This is generally not considered good practice.)

How will our school deal with sexually explicit questions?
Possible statements

Our school will:
* answer all questions asked;
* answer only those questions that relate directly to the agreed programme/lesson;
* make it clear, through ground rules, that nobody should ask personal questions;
* be prepared to modify the programme if a certain question recurs (perhaps because of media coverage);
* use a question box (a box in the classroom to which pupils can 'post' written questions). It will be decided whether or not this question box is anonymous. This box may also be used as a 'buffer' for teachers, if they feel they would like time to consider their answer to a specific question;
* allow individual staff to use their professional judgement to answer questions in front of the whole class or individually;
* encourage pupils to ask their parents/carers any question outside the planned programme;
* with the pupil's permission, inform parents/carers about questions their child has asked;
* make provision for questions about sex, reproduction and puberty to be answered individually, as they arise, outside the planned programme. Parents/carers will be informed of this decision in the school prospectus so that they can exercise their right for this not to happen with their child;
* tell pupils that their question will be answered in a later part of the SRE programme (if necessary).

What kind of language will be considered acceptable and appropriate for use in SRE lessons?
Possible statements
All staff will:
- ★ use the correct terms for all body parts as this is deemed good practice;
- ★ openly teach pupils what 'slang' words mean and that some are offensive;
- ★ avoid the use of any slang.

What ground rules specific to SRE will our junior school use?
Possible statements
- ★ Respect will be shown at all times.
- ★ No personal questions are acceptable in SRE lessons.
- ★ If it is perceived that anyone is at risk from harm, another adult will need to be told.
- ★ Strategies will be developed to ease embarrassment if it occurs.

Single- and mixed-sex groups
Possible statements
- ★ All pupils will learn about both sexes. However, where possible, opportunities will be made for pupils to discuss matters further in single-sex groups or individually.
- ★ All lessons will be taught in mixed-sex groups.
- ★ All lessons will be taught in single-sex groups.

---

j. DISSEMINATION OF THE POLICY
To whom will the policy be available?
Possible statement
All teachers and governors receive a copy of the policy. Training is regularly delivered to staff on policy content. A copy will be provided for parents/carers on request. A short summary of the policy is included in the school prospectus.

How will it be made available?
Possible statement
The PSHE coordinator facilitates the gathering of policy feedback from parents, staff and pupils every two years.

Action plan for SRE overhaul

❶ Carry out a simple audit SRE policy
When was it last updated?
Is it comprehensive enough ? Use the policy guidance on page 21.

Does the SRE programme include a spiral programme that covers:
- ★ growing up and development
- ★ the physical and emotional changes of puberty
- ★ naming sexual organs
- ★ reproduction and sex
- ★ the right you have over your own body
- ★ personal hygiene
- ★ positive body image
- ★ challenging media messages
- ★ accessing help and support
- ★ challenging prejudice?

❷ Get governors involved and aware of SRE issues
- ★ Appoint a governor with responsibilities towards SRE and discuss an SRE overhaul.
- ★ Invite governors to staff SRE training and meetings.

❸ Consultation – involving the whole school community
- ★ Consult parents/carers about SRE – possibly using the questionnaire on page 63.
- ★ Find out what pupils know and want to know via school council discussions, questionnaires, poster making, videos and feedback. Write a pupil-friendly SRE policy (see the ideas on page 64).

❹ Draft a new policy
- ★ Consider the findings from parents/carers and pupils' consultation.
- ★ Make the draft policy available to staff, governors and parents/carers. Invite feedback.

❺ Develop a suggested SRE programme
- ★ Either map PSHE and embed SRE or concentrate on the 'biological' part of SRE as a half-term block in each year group.

❻ Deliver a staff meeting (or two) about SRE. This could:
- ★ use some of the training activities in this book;
- ★ consider the issues found in 'A guide to good practice in SRE' on page 10;
- ★ discuss draft policy;
- ★ use time to look at the suggested programme.

❼ Involve parents/carers – before and during the SRE programme (other than consultation)
- ★ Run a parents'/carers' session (if needed) that aims to make parents/carers supportive of SRE.
- ★ Send out the SRE information leaflet for parents/carers found on pages 76-77. (this addresses commonly cited concerns amongst other things.)
- ★ Send a pre-programme letter (see the example found on page 75) to parents/carers prior to the delivery of the biological programme that reminds them of their right to withdraw their child, outlines the programme and invites them to school to discuss any concerns they might have.
- ★ Set SRE homework that aims to prompt discussions between parents/carers and their children.

❽ Finalise the SRE programme and SRE policy
- ★ Accommodate relevant feedback from staff, governors, pupils and parents/carers.
- ★ Present the documentation to staff and governors.
- ★ Make free copies of the policy available to parents/carers on request.

Puberty and development

TEACHERS' NOTES

The activities on pages 33 to 42 cover aspects of puberty and development. This topic is covered in a variety of ways to provide you with a choice of approaches and so there is enough material to accommodate coverage of this subject in more than one year group or lesson.

What pupils could learn about development and puberty:
★ ★ ★

★ Know how they have changed physically, and with respect to independence and capabilities, since they were a baby and a toddler.

★ Consider what it means to be a grown up.

★ Have a basic knowledge about the changes that happen during puberty.

★ Consider the emotional impact of puberty and explore the feelings that they might have when they anticipate the changes of puberty.

★ Know what periods are and the practicalities of dealing with them.

★ Know that more attention has to be paid to personal hygiene when a person starts the changes of puberty compared with during childhood.

★ Understand that it is always a good idea to talk through any worries they might have with a trusted adult or friend.

★ Know that it is important to be sensitive to others at all times, especially during puberty, and know that it is totally inappropriate to make fun of the changes people experience.

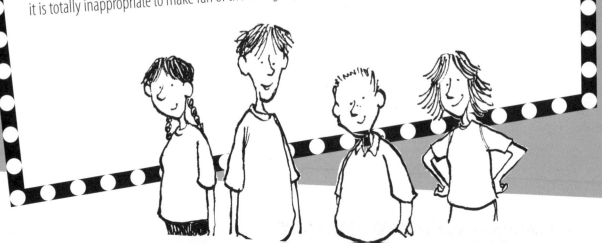

Puberty – what will we look like?

This can be used to introduce the changes of puberty and find out what pupils already know.

Method of delivery

Ask pairs of pupils to look at the sheet and work through the questions. You could ask them to cut out and stick the pictures for a girl and a woman on one sheet of paper, and the boy and a man on another. This will give pupils space to make notes and scribble their answers to the questions around the pictures. The following is a comprehensive list of changes. You could go through all these changes and then ask pupils to add any to their pictures they had not included.

Question 4 can be used to discuss how going through puberty prepares the body for reproduction.

Happens to both boys and girls

- ⚥ Your body has a sudden growth spurt and you can reach a more adult height.
- ⚥ You put on weight.
- ⚥ Your body sweats more.
- ⚥ Your skin and hair can become more greasy.
- ⚥ Your face starts to look more adult.

Happens to boys only

- ♂ Your testicles slowly grow bigger.
- ♂ Your penis slowly grows larger and longer.
- ♂ Hair starts to grow around the base of your penis.
- ♂ Hair grows in your armpits.
- ♂ Your voice becomes deeper. For a while, it can change from deep to squeaky every now and then, but this eventually settles down and your voice remains deep.
- ♂ Your Adam's apple can start to stick out slightly from the front of your neck.
- ♂ Your shoulders and chest grow bigger.
- ♂ You get bigger muscles.
- ♂ You start to grow a moustache, beard and sideburns.
- ♂ You might start to grow hair on your chest.
- ♂ You can have more erections.
- ♂ You can start to ejaculate (when a small amount of sperm comes out of the end of your penis).
- ♂ You can have wet dreams (when sperm comes out from your penis at night).

Happens to girls only

- ♀ Hair starts to grow in the area around the entrance to your vagina — between your legs.
- ♀ A small amount of whitish-yellowish fluid can start to come out of the vagina. This often happens a few months before your periods start.
- ♀ Your hips grow wider and your body begins to have more curves.
- ♀ Hair grows in your armpits.
- ♀ Hair on your arms and legs often grows thicker and longer, and starts to show more.
- ♀ Breasts and nipples slowly grow larger.
- ♀ Your periods (also called menstruation) start.

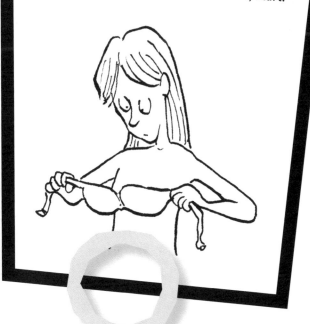

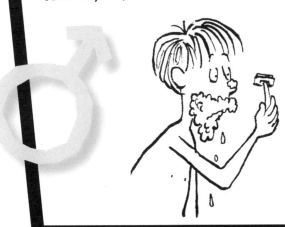

27

Puberty – what's it all about?

Information sheet 1
page 34

This leaflet can be used to introduce pupils to the idea of puberty and some of the changes they will experience.

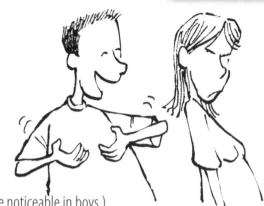

Method of delivery

This can be used as part of a question and answer session or sent home with the pupils to prompt discussion with their parents/carers. You could read through the sheet together and ask the following questions to check for understanding:

❶ What can an adult do that a child cannot? (Reproduce or make babies.)

❷ Do both girls and boys have a growth spurt? (Yes – but it is usually more noticeable in boys.)

❸ What is the earliest age a boy is likely to go through puberty? (Ten)

❹ What other changes do both girls and boys go through? (Hair under arms and between legs, sweat more, greasier skin and hair etc.)

❺ How long can the changes of puberty take? (Two to four years.)

❻ What must you never do to someone who is going through the changes of puberty? (Tease them.)

The changes of puberty

These sentence cards can be used to introduce or consolidate the changes of puberty.

Information sheet 2
page 35

Method of delivery

Ask pupils to sort these sentence cards into three piles headed: 'changes only girls go through', 'changes only boys go through' and 'changes both sexes experience'.

How do I feel about the changes of puberty?

Activity sheet 2
page 36

This activity can be used to explore individual pupil's reactions to the different changes of puberty and to prompt discussions that will hopefully address their concerns.

Method of delivery

This activity is usually best done before any children in the class have begun puberty. Go through each of the changes in the left-hand column and clarify what each thing is. Ask individuals to complete the sheet as honestly as they can. Some guidance to help you to reassure pupils is as follows:

Periods: Periods can take a bit of time to get used to because of the practicalities of dealing with them. However, they soon become a part of life and most girls get used to them relatively quickly.

Wet dreams: (When a boy releases sperm from the end of his penis while he is asleep.) Some boys might feel a bit embarrassed about having made a mess on their pyjamas or sheets. It's best for them not to worry; it is unlikely that whoever washes their sheets will say anything unless they want to talk it through with them.

Body odour: (When someone's body makes a nasty smell – usually because it has not been washed enough.) Every adult sweats but using a deodorant, washing regularly and putting on clean clothes usually means you do not start to smell – so body odour does not have to be part of puberty.

Acne: Not everyone gets acne but most people notice more greasy skin and hair during puberty than in childhood. If acne gets really bad, a doctor can give medical advice that can help.

Wearing a bra: Sometimes other children tease a girl who has started to wear a bra. This is very unkind and should never happen. A girl can wear a bra when she feels she wants to. For some, this is as soon as she starts to develop and, for others, they wait a little longer.

Shaving: At puberty, a boy starts to grow hair on his top lip. This later becomes growth on his chin and sideburns and, eventually, develops into a full beard if he does not shave. It is up to each individual to decide when he wishes to start shaving.

Voice breaking: A boy's voice breaks during puberty as his voice box grows in size. For many boys, their voice changes from being high pitched to low pitched during the voice-breaking process. For some, this lasts for a couple of months but, for others, it can take longer. No one should tease a boy about this as it can make him very self-conscious.

Erections: (When a boy's or man's penis grows stiff because more blood is being pumped into it.) Boys often notice that during puberty they have many more erections than they did as a child. This can make them feel self-conscious – but they do

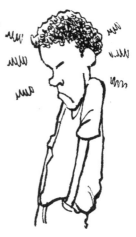

need to remember that they are really likely to be the only person who is aware of it.

Being moody: During puberty, hormones can make some people feel great one minute and terrible the next. It can make them feel really sensitive, self-conscious and emotional. This can also impact on the relationships they have. A person experiencing this can be helped by talking things through with someone they trust and remembering that hormones do eventually settle down.

Developing breasts, growing underarm and pubic hair, growth spurts, looking more adult etc.: Many changes can make a person feel self-conscious and awkward, and nearly everyone going through puberty wonders if they are normal – even though they always are.

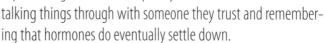

What is a period?

This activity sheet can be used to introduce the idea of periods.

Activity sheet 3
. . . .
page 37

Method of delivery

Read through the sheet with the whole class and discuss the questions below the text. Some guidance for these questions includes:

★ There are girls who start their periods without knowing what is happening to them, so it is not surprising some people know nothing about periods. Some adults find talking about body parts and functions embarrassing and therefore avoid such conversations. Unfortunately, this can leave children not knowing what is going on. You could ask pupils if they think there is anything wrong with knowing this information and discuss their responses.

★ Like all change, periods can take a bit of getting used to. A girl will have to remember to change her sanitary towel regularly and take some spares with her wherever she goes when she has her period.

For extension activities, you could try the following:

★ Have a look at samples of sanitary protection. You could also talk about and/or take a look at tampons as many children may have seen these before and been confused about them. You can explain that older teenagers and women use

tampons and that they soak up the blood before it leaves the body as they are placed inside the hole out of which the blood comes.

★ Discuss how inappropriate it is to tease a girl about periods.

★ Talk about how shy some girls can be about periods and how they like to keep secret the fact that they are having a period. This needs to be respected. However, pupils might like to discuss why they think this is so.

★ Make clear the school's procedure for dealing with a girl who has started her periods at school. Pupils might like to discuss whether this could be changed to make it more discreet if this is what pupils feel is necessary.

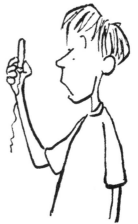

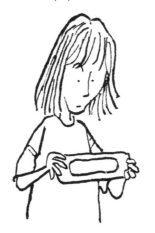

Personal hygiene

Activity sheet 4
page 38

This sheet can be used to introduce the need for increased personal hygiene during puberty.

Method of delivery

Start by talking about what personal hygiene means. With young children, this can mean cleaning teeth twice a day, washing hands before eating, changing clothes every few days, washing hair once or twice a week and changing underwear daily.

Next, introduce the idea that because during puberty we sweat more and our genitals produce fluids that they did not in childhood, we need to take more care over personal hygiene – or we will start to smell. Then ask pupils to work through Question one on the sheet in pairs. Once they have done this, go through their choices one by one as a whole class. Then ask pairs of pupils to have a go at Question two. This consolidates what they have learnt.

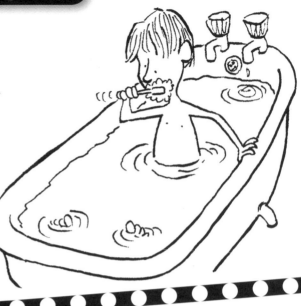

Activity sheet 5
page 39

Being sensitive to others

This sheet explores the idea that a person can become extremely self-conscious during puberty and that it is totally inappropriate to tease someone about their physical appearance or about any of the changes of puberty.

Method of delivery

Read through part one as a whole class and ask pairs of pupils to discuss their answers to the questions. Explain that the green spot would probably make you feel self-conscious. Being self-conscious is when you lack confidence because you are worried about what you look like and whether anyone is going to notice or make a comment.

Next, read the paragraph about puberty and ask pairs to discuss Questions 2 to 4. Ask them to feedback to the class. Hopefully, pupils will have concluded that:

★ It is best to only give positive comments about a person's appearance.

★ No one should ever tease someone about their physical appearance.

★ It is never good to bring another person's physical appearance to other people's attention as this can increase self-consciousness.

★ If a person is the first or last to go through puberty, they can be reassured that everyone does eventually go through it.

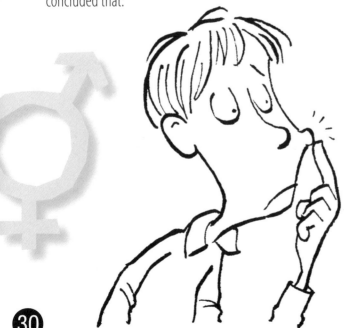

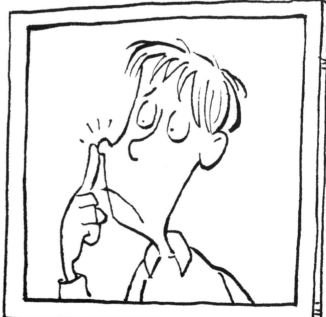

Babies

Activity sheet 6
page 40

This sheet takes a simple look at what babies can do and how children still have some dependence on their parents/carers but not as much as a baby does.

Method of delivery

Ask pupils to consider the two questions on the sheet and complete them in pairs. Highlight how dependent a baby is but how much less dependent a child is. This could lead to discussions about how independence increases with age. Pupils could consider the questions in the box on the right to help with this.

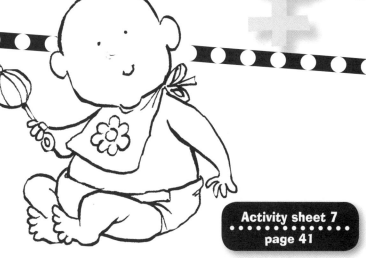

❶ Why are babies so dependent on their parents/carers? (They do not have the skills or knowledge to do things for themselves.)

❷ What kind of things are you still dependent on your parents/carers for? (Food, housing, washing etc.)

❸ What do your parents/carers do to encourage you to be independent? (Show you how to do things safely, encourage you to have a go on your own etc.)

❹ Why is it important that you become more and more independent as you grow up? (You won't live with your parents/carers forever so you need to learn to be self-reliant and be able to do things for yourself.)

What do babies do?

This sheet looks at babies: their development, their dependence and the extensive role of parents/carers.

Method of delivery

The lesson could start with a discussion about any younger brothers or sisters the pupils may have and their memories of what it was like when they were a baby.

Activity sheet 7
page 41

❶ In pairs, pupils could try to put the activities in the order (shown here) that babies start to do them.

smile	6 weeks
hold things	3 months
start to eat mashed-up food	4 months
be able to see a person across a room	5 months
sit up alone	6 months
crawl	9 months
walk	1 year
start to say their first words	1 ½ years

(All of these are very approximate)

❷ Pupils might conclude that it is because a baby can do so little for themselves and they can come to harm as they do not have the ability to know what is dangerous.

❸ Pupils will probably come up with a list of things like pull things down onto themselves, put fingers in sockets, fall down the stairs, swallow things, cut themselves on sharp edges etc.

❹ Answers may include feed them, give them drinks, change their nappies, wash them, carry them, push them in a pushchair, clothe them, entertain them, protect them from the cold/sun, put them to bed etc.

❺ Answers may include cold, hot, hungry, bored, tired, teething, feeling unwell, thirsty, wanting to be picked up, wanting company, frustration because they cannot reach something etc.

❻ Pupils can write a long list here – from being able to read to being able to skateboard!

❼ Lots of this equipment is about keeping the baby safe or helping the parent/carer to look after the baby because it cannot sit up, walk, go to the toilet or eat properly etc.

❽ Pupils might conclude that having a baby too young might stop you getting the job you want, or you might not want to be tied to looking after a baby as you might miss out on the fun of socialising etc. However, having a baby quite early in adulthood might mean you have more energy for the baby and still be quite young when the baby has grown up and left home. Pupils might decide that having a baby when you are quite old might mean that you are not as energetic as you were when you were younger but that you might make wiser decisions about bringing up the child. It's open to discussion. Pupils could vote on it!

Growing up

This sheet covers development and how a person's capabilities improve as they grow up.

Method of delivery

❶ Ask pupils to consider the pictures and, in small groups, try to order them from youngest to oldest. (Point out that it is the baby we are considerng at in the picture where a mother is breastfeeding.) The correct order is: F, D, C, A, H, E, G, B.

F – small baby wrapped up, breastfeeding – probably around two or three months old.

D – baby rolling around (cannot crawl yet), grabbing toes – probably about four or five months old.

C – baby sitting up – probably six to eight months old.

A – baby crawling – probably about nine months old.

H – toddler walking – probably 12 months old.

E – little girl of about three or four years old sitting on the floor playing with toys

G – boy cycling –about six or seven years old.

B – teenager on a skateboard.

Ask pupils what made them decide on the order they chose. Next, ask pupils to work through Questions 2 to 4. Encourage them to produce the longest lists they can for Questions 3 and 4. Here are some possible answers to the questions:

❷ The order is: grab things, sit up, crawl, walk, speak, run and ride a bike.

❸ Depending on the age of the children, their answers might include: draw, run, understand words, speak, use a knife and fork, go to the toilet independently, go to bed, clean teeth, write, use scissors, ride a bike, swim etc.

❹ Answers could include: drive, earn money, have children, buy a house, drink alcohol, cook meals, leave the house on their own, vote etc.

As an extension activity, pupils could cut out toys from a catalogue and order them to show the stages of children's development.

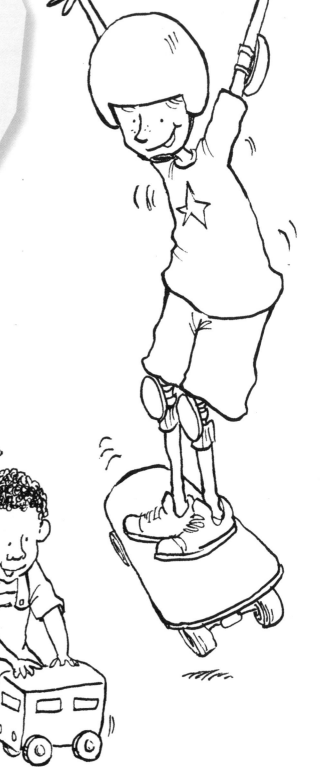

Puberty – what will we look like?

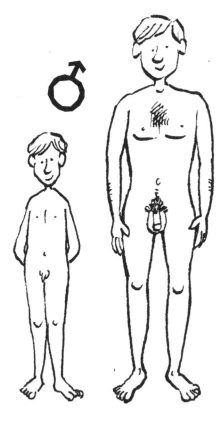

Puberty is a time when we change from being a child to being a young adult. This happens at slightly different times for different people. It often starts between the ages of 10 and 14 but can sometimes be earlier or later.

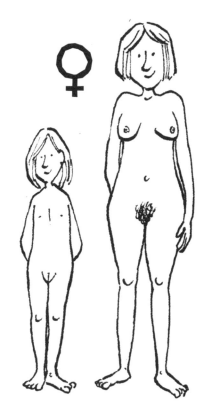

❶ Look at the pictures above that show how a boy has changed to a man and a girl to a woman. Circle the main changes you can see.

❷ List as many changes as you can think of that happen to girls during puberty.

_____

_____

_____

❸ List as many changes as you can think of that happen to boys during puberty.

_____

_____

_____

❹ List as many changes as you can think of that happen to both girls and boys during puberty.

_____

_____

_____

❺ Why do you think these changes happen?

_____

_____

_____

Activity sheet 1 * SRE 7–9   © Molly Potter 2009

Puberty – what's it all about?

Puberty is the name given to the time when a child's body grows into an adult's body. Obviously adults are bigger than children but growing is not the only change to happen. Male and female bodies change during puberty so they can eventually make babies.

Don't worry though: these changes don't happen overnight. You don't go to bed a child and wake up an adult! It can take between two and four years for all the changes to happen.

Boys

Boys tend to start puberty later than girls. Some boys might start puberty as young as ten but others might not start until they are about 15. The age that puberty starts has no effect on what the man ends up looking like.

Here are some of the main changes boys go through during puberty:
- ♂ grow much taller in a short time
- ♂ voice becomes deep
- ♂ penis and testicles grow bigger
- ♂ grow hair around their penis and testicles
- ♂ grow hair in their armpits
- ♂ hair starts to grow on their face
- ♂ muscles get bigger
- ♂ hair and skin becomes greasier
- ♂ sweat more
- ♂ start to make sperm

Girls

Girls usually start puberty between the ages of 8 and As with boys, the age that a girl starts puberty has no effect on what she will end up looking like as an adult.

Here are some of the main changes a girl goes through during puberty:
- ♀ grow much taller in a short time
- ♀ grow hair in their armpits
- ♀ grow hair between their legs
- ♀ hair and skin becomes greasier
- ♀ sweat more
- ♀ breasts start to grow
- ♀ hips get wider
- ♀ periods start

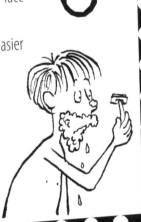

Change

Puberty can sometimes feel like it is a lot to get used to – like with all change. It always helps if you have someone to talk to and ask questions about it. Also, remember that everyone goes through puberty, so don't make anyone feel self-conscious by teasing them about the changes they are going through - that would be very unkind.

Information sheet 1   SRE 7–9   © Molly Potter 2009

The changes of puberty

Puberty is a time when we change from being a child to being a young adult.

This happens at slightly different times for different people.

It often starts between the ages of 10 and 14 but

can sometimes be earlier or later.

Periods start	You grow taller
You eat more	You may start to fancy people
Hair and skin may become more greasy	Breasts develop
Penis and testicles get bigger	Wet dreams might happen
Pubic hair starts to grow between your legs	Your voice gets deeper
You sweat more	Spots may appear
You start to grow hair under your arms	Hair grows on your face
You can have mood swings	Hips become wider
Vaginal discharge (small amount of sticky white fluid) occurs	Sperm are made

Information sheet 2   SRE 7–9   © Molly Potter 2009

How do I feel about the changes of puberty?

	yucky	OK	great	scary	embarrassing	uncomfortable	awkward	grown up
periods								
developing breasts								
wet dreams								
pubic hair								
body odour								
underarm hair								
acne (spots)								
wearing a bra								
shaving								
erections								
voice breaking								
being moody								
greasy hair								
growth spurt								
look like an adult								

Activity sheet 2 * SRE 7–9 © Molly Potter 2009

What is a period?

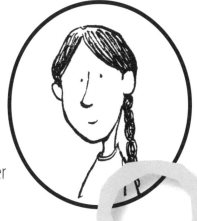

When a girl grows up, she will start her periods.

This sheet explains what a period is.

When a girl starts her periods, the first thing she will notice is a little blood in her knickers. At first this is often brown.

At this point, she will probably need to tell someone, like her mum, dad or a teacher, so that she can be helped.

The blood that dribbles out from a hole between a girl's legs is soaked up using protection called a sanitary towel. This is like a cotton wool pad that is stuck in the knickers. These are bought from shops – usually by a girl's family. Schools usually have some for girls who start their periods at school.

The girl will need to change the towel about four times a day.

When a girl needs to get rid of the towel, she can put it in the bins (that are often blue or brown) found in the girls' toilets – next to the actual toilet.

A girl only loses a few spoonfuls of blood in about four to six days – which is how long a period usually lasts. She usually has a period once a month.

A girl's periods usually start a while after her breasts have started to grow. Most girls start at about 12 years of age but some start as young as 8 or 9, and some start when they are 15 or 16.

❶ Did you know what periods were before you read this and, if you did, who told you about them?

_____

_____

❷ When a girl starts her periods, she has to get used to using sanitary towels. Do you think this might be difficult and, if so, why?

_____

_____

_____

Activity sheet 3 * SRE 7–9   © Molly Potter 2009

Personal hygiene

When a child reaches puberty, they need to take more care with keeping clean, or they may start to smell.

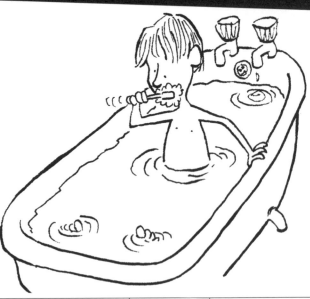

❶ Which of the following pieces of advice do you think a teenager needs to take and which do you think they could ignore? Tick the correct box.

Advice for someone once they reach puberty	Take this advice	Ignore this advice
It is a good idea to take a shower at least once a day because you sweat a lot more than when you were a child.		
Putting on lots of layers of clothing will stop you from getting smelly.		
You might need to start washing your hair a bit more than when you were a child because it gets greasier.		
You do not need to clean your teeth at all during puberty.		
When you have a bath, put some sugar in it to make you sweeter.		
It is a good idea to start using deodorant at puberty.		
It's OK to wear the same socks all week as long as they are yellow.		
Always take an umbrella into the shower.		
You definitely need to put on new underpants/knickers every day.		
If you do some sport and get really hot and sweaty, it's a good idea to take a shower afterwards.		
If your feet start to smell cheesy, make sure everyone smells them.		
You need to put clean clothes on every day — if you wear the same clothes you wore yesterday, you are likely to get a bit smelly.		
Only use soap in January.		

❷ Draw a picture on the back of this sheet (no words) that could be used to help you to explain to an alien what each of the following are. See if a partner can match your pictures to the correct activity!

Use deodorant	Clean teeth	Take a shower or have a bath
Put on clean clothes	Wash hair	Use soap and shampoo
Put on clean underpants every day	Comb hair	

Activity sheet 4 * SRE 7–9   © Molly Potter 2009

Being sensitive to others

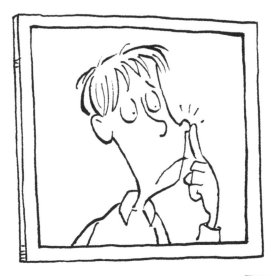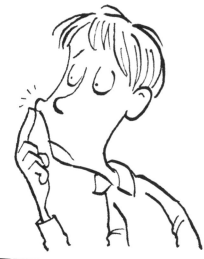

1 Imagine if one day you looked in the mirror and noticed that you had grown a huge, green spot on your cheek. This is a spot that just could not be removed, hidden or covered up. With a partner, discuss the questions on the right.

★ How would this make you feel?
★ What would you think?
★ What would you want to do?
★ How would you want others to treat you when they saw the spot?

Read this short paragraph:

During puberty, our bodies change a lot. Some of these changes can make us feel self-conscious – as if we had woken up with a bright green spot on our face. Because our bodies have changed, we can also start to wonder if we are normal or not.

2 Imagine you were the very first person in your class to start puberty. With a partner, discuss the questions on the right.

3 Imagine you were the very last person in your class to start puberty. With a partner, discuss the questions on the right.

★ How do you think this would make you feel?

★ What is the worst thing a friend could do or say to you?

★ How would you like people to behave when they noticed that your body was starting to change?

4 What do you think are the dos and don'ts of supporting someone who is going through puberty?

Activity sheet 5 * SRE 7–9   © Molly Potter 2009

Babies

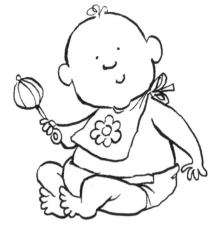 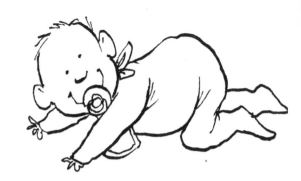

❶ Circle the things a baby can do:

speak   cry   smile   run   move

ride a bike   count   catch a ball   eat   wash

shake a rattle   get dressed   drink   write

❷ Which of these things do your parents or carers still have to do for you? Put a tick (√) or cross (x) in each box.

	Do they do this for you now?	Will they continue to do this for you when you are a grown up?
Change your nappy		
Carry you around		
Keep you safe		
Feed you		
Give you drinks		
Dress you		
Wash you		
Brush your teeth		
Love you		

Activity sheet 6 * SRE 7–9 © Molly Potter 2009

What do babies do?

❶ See if you can match up what a baby can do (on the left) with the age at which he or she can do it (on the right)! (The ages are not exactly true for all babies as they are all different.)

be able to see a person across a room	**6 weeks**
smile	**3 months**
start to say their first words	**4 months**
hold things	**5 months**
crawl	**6 months**
start to eat mashed-up food	**9 months**
sit up alone	**1 year**
walk	**1½ years**

❷ Babies need a lot of care. Why do you think this is?

_____

_____

❸ If a baby who can crawl was left on his or her own, what dangerous things might happen?

_____

_____

❹ Make a list of all the things a mother, father or carer has to do for a baby.

_____

_____

❺ All babies cry! For what reasons do you think a baby cries?

_____

_____

❻ What things can you do now that you could not do as a one year old?

_____

_____

❼ Think of all the equipment people use to help them to look after a baby. Why is this equipment needed?

_____

_____

❽ At what age do you think it is a good idea for a person to start having babies? Why?

_____

_____

Growing up

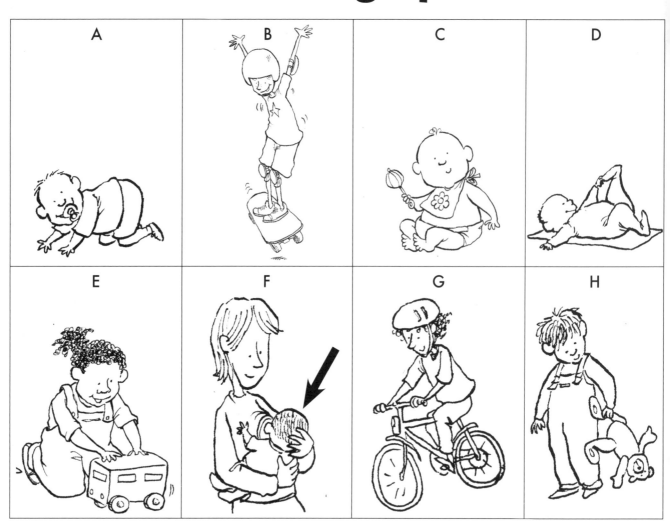

❶ Order these people from the youngest to the oldest. Write the letters in the correct order in the spaces below.

Youngest _____   _____   _____   _____   _____   _____   _____   _____ Oldest

❷ In what order do we learn to do the following things?

Write the answers in the correct order underneath.

walk	speak	grab things	ride a bike	run	sit up	crawl

1st _____   2nd _____   3rd _____   4th _____

5th _____   6th _____   7th _____

❸ What things can you do now that you could not do when you were a baby?

_____

❹ What things will you be able to do as an adult that you cannot do now?

_____

Activity sheet 8   SRE 7–9   © Molly Potter 2009

Reproduction, sex and life cycles

TEACHERS' NOTES

The activities on pages 46 to 51 cover aspects of reproduction, sex and life cycles.

These topics are covered in a variety of ways to provide you with a choice of

approaches and so there is enough material to accommodate different teaching

styles and coverage of this subject in more than one year group or lesson.

What pupils could learn about reproduction, sex and life cycles
★ ★ ★

★ Know the basic stages of the human life cycle.
★ Consider the responsibilities of being a parent/carer.
★ Know the main external physical differences between a male and a female.
★ Know which parts of the body are responsible for making a baby.
★ Be introduced to the basics of reproduction and sex.
★ Know some information about pregnancy and birth.

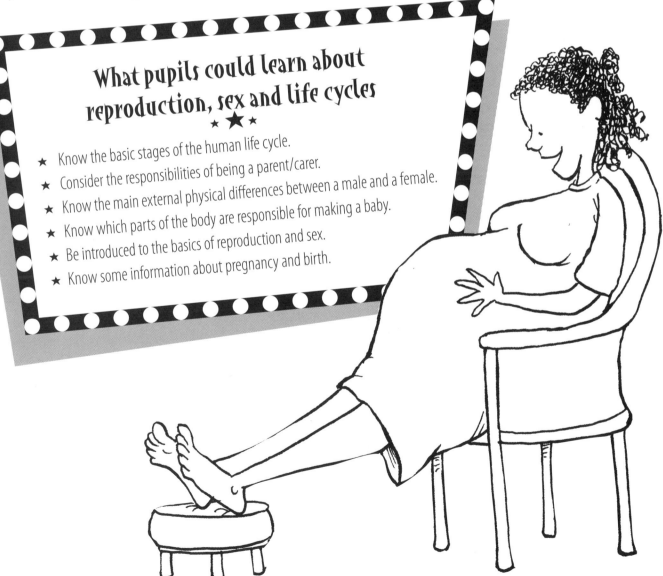

The human life cycle

This considers the main features of the human life cycle.

Method of delivery

This lesson is best carried out as a discussion with bits of scrap paper so pupils can note down any points they make. Notice that death has been omitted from the life cycle. As a teacher, you will probably be aware of any sensitivity to the topic of death, and so it is up to you whether or not you decide to include it.

There are numerous extension activities, particularly for the younger children, such as making a life stages booklet (including what people are capable of at the different stages) or collecting magazine pictures of the different stages. Pupils could also consider which stage people they know are at. With Question 7, pupils need to be challenged about any prejudices they might express, as older people can be fit and capable to their dying day — although pupils' descriptions of their own grandparents will hopefully show that old people vary as much as anyone else!

Activity sheet 1
page 46

Parents and carers

This looks at the roles and responsibilities of parents and carers.

Method of delivery

This can be mostly a discussion activity, with paper available for Questions 3 and 10.

★ Pupils need to be aware of the supportive aspects of being a parent or carer as well as the physical tasks that come with parenthood.

★ In discussing why people choose to be parents, it needs to be emphasised that children can bring a lot of joy to their parents and carers! Pupils could think about why this is.

★ Pupils also need to consider that parents/carers are human (!) and do have moods, make mistakes, get exhausted and don't always get it 'right'.

★ If time allows, pupils could act out a conflict between a child and a parent to consider the following questions:

❶ Why was there an argument? What was it really about?

❷ How was the child feeling?

❸ What was the parent/carer feeling?

❹ How could the argument be sorted so that both child and parent are happy?

Activity sheet 2
page 47

Males and females

This sheet highlights that males and females have different body parts and that adults have some features that children do not have.

Activity sheet 3
page 48

Method of delivery

Show pupils the sheet and ask them to label all the body parts listed. Make it clear that if everyone has a particular feature (e.g. a navel), then the labels need to show this. Once pupils have completed the sheet, go through the answers.

Body parts needed to make a baby

Activity sheet 4
page 49

This sheet explains the body parts involved in sex and reproduction, and how a baby is made. Pupils can fill in the missing words on the sheet.

Method of delivery

Hand the sheet out so pupils can look at the pictures. Explain to pupils what each of the words at the top of the sheet means:
Penis: sometimes called a 'willy'. It's what a boy and man uses to pee.
Vagina: a hole or tube that has its entrance between a girl or woman's legs. It is the hole from which babies come out.
Womb: the place inside a woman where a baby grows.
Eggs: are found inside a woman. They are tiny. Together with a sperm from a man, they can make a baby.

★ Ask pupils if they know why a child can look a bit like both their mother and father. Clear up any misunderstandings and explain that a baby starts to grow when an egg from the mother and sperm from the father join together. Explain that this happens inside the mother.

★ Ask pupils where a baby grows. Explain that a baby starts as a tiny dot of a few cells and that this grows in the mother's tummy. Tell the pupils that it takes about nine months for the baby to grow from these tiny cells to a baby big enough to be born.

★ Ask pupils how they think the baby gets out of the mother. Explain that the baby is born out of the mother's vagina. Some pupils may know some details about their births that they might like to share with the class.

Sex and how babies are made

Activity sheet 5
page 50

This sheet can be used to consolidate knowledge about sexual reproduction.

Method of delivery

Ask pairs of pupils to work through the sheet and decide if each statement is true or false. Once they have completed the sheet, go through the answers and respond to any questions the pupils might have.

Some guidance on the answers:

1 True – well you certainly need sperm that comes from men and an egg that comes from a woman.

2 False.

3 True.

4 No, sperm look like tiny tadpoles. They are too small to be seen without a microscope. A woman's egg is about the size of a full stop.

5 True.

6 True.

7 False – children often believe this because sexual intercourse is most commonly taught in terms of reproduction. You can explain that a man and a woman (and two women, and two men) can have sex because it's a kind of sharing; it feels nice and can make people feel very close.

8 True – they move about so that the penis slides partially in and out of the vagina and this feels nice for both the man and the woman.

9 True.

10 False – during sex, sperm comes out of the end of a man's penis into the woman's vagina. These sperm travel up inside the woman and if she has an egg ready, a baby can start to grow in her womb.

11 False – they are tiny and you would need a powerful microscope to see them.

12 False – because a woman only has an egg ready for a short while each month and because men and women can use contraception, which stops a baby from growing. Condoms are one kind of contraception that lots of people have heard of. They work by covering the penis and preventing the sperm from getting inside the woman.

13 False – babies take about nine months to grow inside a woman.

14 False – being born can take hours (sometimes even a couple of days). It can be a lot of hard work and often causes pain for the woman. The baby is born out of the vagina unless the baby is born by caesarean section. This is another normal way for a baby to be born. A caesarean birth is when a mother has an operation to have her baby born directly from the womb through a hole cut by a surgeon. The mother feels nothing when this happens as she is given an anaesthetic.

15 True – talking about sex and body parts is not something everyone is comfortable with. This is why it is never good to ask personal questions about sex.

Pregnancy, babies & birth – make it true

This sheet could be used to introduce or revise some of the main features about pregnancy, babies and birth.

Method of delivery

Ask pairs of pupils to go through the sheet to see if they can work out which word in each sentence needs to be replaced and what it needs to be replaced with. After a while, go through the answers (that follow) and respond to any questions the pupils might have.

Activity sheet 6
page 51

Answers to the questions:

1 Change rabbit to baby

2 Change smiles to grows

3 Change eyes to legs

4 Change coat to belly

5 Change father to mother

6 Change eat to weigh

7 Change weeks to hours

8 Change painted to born

9 Change three to two

10 Change bread to milk

11 Change stripy to no

12 Change hear to feel

13 Change can to can't

14 Change ski to (move, sneeze, feed, blink etc.)

The human life cycle

This is the order of a human life:

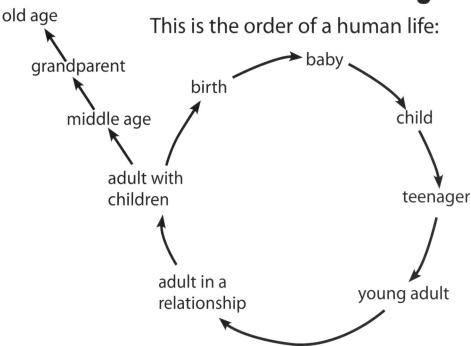

Now answer the following questions.

❶ Why is it called a life 'cycle'?

_____

❷ Not everyone follows this route through life. List as many ways as you can think of to show how a life can be different from this particular route.

_____

_____

_____

❸ Where on this cycle are you likely to be when you are the following ages?

2_____ 10_____ 15 _____

40_____ 70_____

❹ At which stage would you be most likely to do the following things?

Learn to drive _____

Learn to speak _____

Go to school _____

Get a boyfriend or girlfriend _____

Get a job _____

❺ List as many things as you can think of that you can do as a child that you couldn't do as a baby.

_____

_____

_____

❻ List as many things as you can think of that you get better at as you change from a child to a young adult. _____

_____

❼ How do you think people change when they move from middle age to old age?_____

_____

❽ What do you think are likely to be the best things about growing up? _____

_____

❾ What do you think you will miss about being a child?_____

_____

_____

Activity sheet 1 * SRE 7–9   © Molly Potter 2009

Parents and carers

Read the advert and discuss these questions with a partner.

❶ Would you do this job?

❷ Why do you think people choose to do this job?

❸ In an average week, what tasks do your parents/carers do? Create a list and make it as long as you can.

❹ What type of personality do you think makes a good parent/carer?

❺ Sometimes our parents/carers don't let us do what we want to. Why do you think this is?

❻ Sometimes our parents/carers get cross with us and tell us off. Why do you think this is?

❼ What do you think your parent/carer would say are the good things about being a parent/carer?

❽ What rules do your parents/carers have for you? Think about each rule. Is it there to keep you safe, to make you a better person, to keep you healthy or to make you considerate towards others?

❾ What do you think your parents/carers hope that you will do in your life?

❿ Re-write the advert on the back of this sheet but this time make the job sound fantastic — but don't lie!

Activity sheet 2 * SRE 7–9   © Molly Potter 2009

Males and females

Males are men and boys. Females are women and girls.

Do males or females (or both) have the following body parts?

Label the body parts on these pictures. Note that both the adult and child have some things and only the adult has other things. Show this with your labels.

navel   penis   pubic hair   arms   chest hair   beard

vagina   clitoris   breasts   nipples   testicles   underarm hair

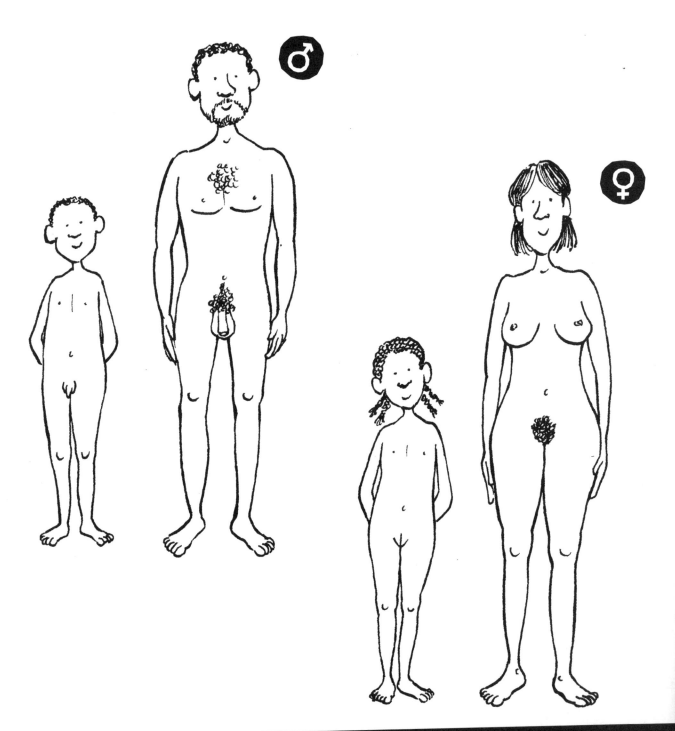

Activity sheet 3   SRE 7–9   © Molly Potter 2009

Body parts needed to make a baby

Write the correct words into the spaces below.

Cross them off the list as you use them.

sperm   penis   vagina   penis   womb   sperm   eggs   vagina

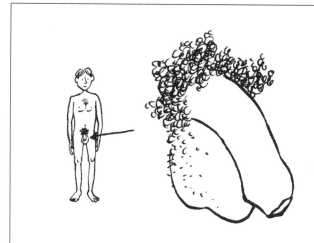

A man has a _____.

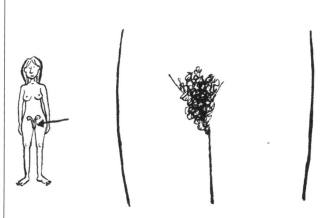

A woman has a _____.
This is a hole that has an entrance between a woman's legs.

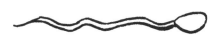

A man has _____. They are tiny.
Only one is needed to make a baby but many can come out of the man's penis.

A woman has _____. She makes them inside her.
Only one is needed to make a baby. They are the size of a full stop.

To make a baby, the man puts his _____ inside the woman's vagina. This is called sex and it feels nice for the adults.

When the man and woman have sex, _____ comes out of the end of the man's penis. It goes inside the woman and if she has an egg ready, a baby can start to grow.

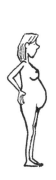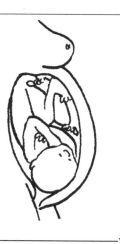

A baby grows in a woman's _____.

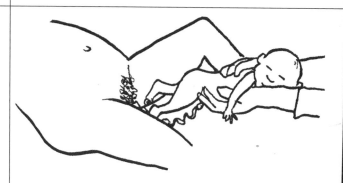

The baby is most often born out of the mummy's _____.

Sex and how babies are made

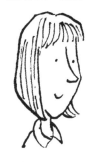
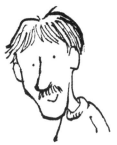

Answer the following
questions. Circle true or false.

1 You need both a man and a woman to make a baby. True or False

2 A baby is made when a man and a woman drink strawberry milkshake together. True or False

3 A baby can start to grow when a sperm from a man and an egg from a woman join together. True or False

4 Sperm look like tiny octopuses. True or False

5 The sperm need to get inside a woman to make a baby. True or False

6 The sperm go inside a woman when the man and woman have sex. True or False

7 A man and a woman only ever have sex when they want to make a baby. True or False

8 Sexual intercourse or sex is when a man puts his penis inside a woman's vagina. True or False

9 A man's penis is sometimes called a 'willy' but different families have different names for this body part. True or False

10 During sex, sperm comes out of the man's ears. True or False

11 Sperm are the size of apples. True or False

12 A woman gets pregnant every time she has sex. True or False

13 A baby grows for just two weeks inside the mother's womb and then it is ready to be born. True or False

14 When a baby is ready to be born, it shouts 'I'm ready' and pops out of the mother's vagina. True or False

15 Some adults are shy when it comes to talking about sex. True or False

Activity sheet 5   SRE 7–9   © Molly Potter 2009

Pregnancy, babies and birth – make it true

All of these statements are false. Change just one word in each to make them all true. The first one has been done for you.

---

❶ It takes nine months to grow a rabbit in a woman's womb (tummy).

Change _____ rabbit _____

To _____ baby _____

---

❷ The baby starts tiny but then smiles inside the womb until it is big enough to be born.

Change _____

To _____

---

❸ A baby is born out of its mummy's vagina (a hole between her eyes).

Change _____

To _____

---

❹ A person's coat button is where they were attached to their mummy when they were inside the womb.

Change _____

To _____

---

❺ Inside the womb a baby gets its food from its father.

Change _____

To _____

---

❻ When babies are first born, they eat about 3 kilograms.

Change _____

To _____

---

❼ It can take a mother several weeks to push a baby out.

Change _____

To _____

---

❽ Most babies are painted in hospital.

Change _____

To _____

---

❾ Twins are made when three babies grow inside the womb at the same time.

Change _____

To _____

---

❿ A mum's breasts make bread that can feed a baby after it is born.

Change _____

To _____

⓫ When a baby is first born, it has stripy clothes on.

Change _____

To _____

⓬ A mum can hear her baby kick her when it is inside her womb.

Change _____

To _____

⓭ A baby can walk just after it is born.

Change _____

To _____

⓮ A newborn baby can cry and ski.

Change _____

To _____

Activity sheet 6   SRE 7–9   © Molly Potter 2009

Other related topics

TEACHERS' NOTES
Keeping safe

Activity sheet 1
page 54

This covers the right everyone has not to receive unwelcome touching of any kind. Although this lesson does not explicitly cover sexual abuse, it spells out a child's rights in a way that will help pupils to understand that sexual abuse is wrong should they ever tragically encounter it. This sheet also considers the support networks a child could turn to for help.

Method of delivery

Ask pairs of pupils to discuss the scenarios on the sheet. There could be some debate where one pupil might be happy to receive a particular touch that another pupil might not be happy with (e.g. a teacher ruffling hair). There might also be debate about how sometimes it might feel OK and other times it might not, depending on the person and the situation. This is fine as the whole point is that you do not have to put up with touching of any kind – whenever it is or feels unwelcome. This includes touching that just makes you feel a bit uncomfortable. Explain that everyone needs to respect other people's personal space and to understand that some types of touching can be unwelcome to some individuals. Tell the pupils that it is usually good practice to ask a person before you touch them. For example, if an adult was teaching a new sport and needed to touch someone to show them how to position themselves, they would usually ask permission before doing so. Next, complete the second part of the sheet where pupils identify their support networks. Stress the need to keep telling adults until someone helps, as in the worst case scenarios (e.g. sexual or physical abuse), many children stop asking for help (if they ask at all) perhaps because they feel their situation is all their fault. One adult ignoring their request for help is a knockback that could prevent them from asking another adult, unless it has been emphasised to them to persist for help.

***Note:* There is a slim chance that a lesson like this can cause a disclosure that could be a child protection situation. Be sure to have a clear understanding of your school's safeguarding children policy.**

What is so important about looking good?

This sheet challenges the notion that the most important thing about a person is what they look like.

Activity sheet 2
page 55

Method of delivery

Ask pairs of pupils to discuss questions 1 to 5. Then go through the questions as a class with the following in mind:

★ With the way the media constantly present us with 'good-looking' celebrities and models, it is easy to assume that what a person looks like is the most important thing about them. Believing this idea can make people feel bad about themselves.

★ Attractiveness is not just about what we look like. There are many qualities that a person can have that can make them attractive e.g. confidence, optimism, helpfulness, kindness, being witty or funny, being a good listener, telling interesting stories etc.

★ People generally become more attractive to others the more familiar they become.

★ Some people become obsessed with looking good which cannot be very good their well-being and must also be time consuming.

Note: **While you don't want to give the message that being good-looking is a bad thing, you need to craft discussion to counter the idea that what you look like is the most important thing about a person.**

Next, ask pupils to use the main messages that they have received from the discussion to complete Question 6 on the sheet in pairs.

What do we think about girls and boys?

This explores how girls and boys perceive each other and can be used to challenge any sexual stereotyping pupils carry out.

Method of delivery

Where possible, ask mixed-sex pairs of pupils to discuss and complete the grid and then answer questions 2 and 3.

Some guidance about each section:

Toys: toys marketed at girls tend to be pink, are about modelling the role of a homekeeper and are 'gentle' and toys marketed at boys tend to be geared to action, adventure, being tough and are modelled towards activities traditionally seen as male (e.g. using tools). Ask pupils if there is anything wrong with girls playing with boys' toys and boys playing with girls' toys.

Girls/boys when they play together: pupils might consider that girls talk more than boys, that boys play more rough and energetic games than girls, that boys like to play-fight more than girls etc. Ask pupils if these statements are true of all girls and all boys and if it matters if a girl likes physical games and a boy likes to sit down and chat.

How girls/boys behave in lessons: pupils might tend to think that girls concentrate more than boys, boys are more disorganised and messy than girls, boys like Science and girls like Art etc. Point out that this is not true of all boys and all girls.

What boys/girls must never do or people might laugh at them: this prompt needs careful handling. Pupils might conclude that if a girl behaves in a way that is traditionally seen as male behaviour, this is OK (she is a tomboy). However, if a girl is aggressive, this tends to be less acceptable than if a boy is. Pupils might also conclude that if a boy behaves in a way that is traditionally seen as female behaviour, some people might make fun of him. This needs to be challenged. Is there anything wrong with a boy playing with dolls or not liking sport?

Next, open up the discussion to the whole class by brainstorming 'boys' and 'girls' on the board and seeing what ideas the pupils produced using the grids on the sheet. Continue to challenge any sexual stereotyping that girls or boys suggest about their own or the opposite sex. For example, if someone says, 'Boys run around and are really active', ask pupils if girls can do that too.

Close the lesson by consolidating the idea that if anyone behaves in a way that does not harm anyone but that is a little different from most people, we need to celebrate the fact they are different and applaud their courage in not going along with the crowd.

Activity sheet 3
page 56

Family

Activity sheet 4
page 57

This sheet unpicks what is meant by 'family' and explores diversity in family set-ups.

Method of delivery

You could start the lesson by asking pupils to draw a family to see what they produce and consider how their ideas vary. Then read through the sheet and allow pupils to discuss the questions. Here are some discussion prompts for the questions:

❶ Your family are there for you, you feel part of a family, it's where you feel safe and secure, they are people that support you etc. Different pupils will feel differently towards their families.

❷ Provide a home, food, love, support, help you to learn, take you to places etc.

❸ Answers will vary considerably. Examples include: sit down to meals, visit places, celebrate birthdays etc.

❹ and ❺ Pupils will express a variety of views.

❻ Encourage pupils to be realistic. If they include rules like 'make all meals ice-cream', discuss why this would not be a good idea and why most parents/carers would not let this happen. Rules could include things like: love your children, forgive your children for making mistakes, be consistent, don't have favourites, spend time with your children, be interested in the things your children are interested in etc.

Pupils could then try to create a list as long as they can from the sentence start: 'A family...'.

Keeping safe

❶ Which of these do you think you would like, not mind, not like or feel uncomfortable about?

Another child punching you while you were in a queue waiting to go into assembly.

A friend giving you a hug because you were upset.

Your mum/dad/carer giving you a hug because you gave them a present.

Someone in the park that you did not know running up to you and kissing you on the cheek.

A friend shaking your hand to make a deal about something.

A friend of your parents or carers putting their hand on your bottom.

An adult you hardly knew putting their arm round you when you were walking home from school.

A toddler that you know holding your hand so they can cross the road safely.

A teacher ruffling your hair because you had just done something really funny.

A babysitter that you had never met before trying to get you to sit on their lap.

If anyone touches you in a way you do not like, you have the right to stop it from happening.

If telling the person to stop touching you does not prevent it from happening, you need to find an adult you trust to tell. If that adult does nothing to help, you need to find another adult to tell. You need to keep telling until someone helps. This is true of any situation that happens where you feel you cannot sort it out on your own.

❷ List five adults who you would ask for help if you needed it.

Activity sheet 1 * SRE 7–9   © Molly Potter 2009

What is so important about looking good?

Discuss these questions with a partner. Make some notes.

1 Do you think it is more important that a cake looks good or tastes good?

2 Would you rather have a toy kept in a glass case (to keep it looking new) that you could only look at or a toy you could play with?

3 Do you think that if a person looks like a model from a magazine, they are definitely going to be a kind or interesting person?

4 Would you rather have a friend that:

wore great trainers	OR	was good at making you laugh?	
always wore trendy clothes	OR	was always willing to help you?	
fussed about keeping their hair neat	OR	was adventurous?	
had loads of different outfits	OR	was generous?	
always looked perfect	OR	was interesting to talk to?	

Here are some proverbs that relate to beauty.

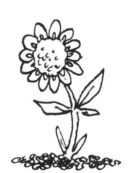

- **Beauty is only skin deep.**
  Traditional proverb
- **Beauty is in the eye of the beholder.**
  English proverb
- **One cannot make soup out of beauty.**
  Estonian proverb
- **Charm is stronger than beauty.**
  Maltese proverb
- **If there is character, ugliness becomes beauty; if there is none, beauty becomes ugliness.**
  Nigerian proverb
- **Beauty without wisdom is like a flower in the mud.**
  Romanian proverb

5 What message is each proverb giving you?

6 On a separate piece of paper, design an advert that tries to sell one of the following messages:

★ Your personality is more important than what you look like.

★ It is not good to think that what a person looks like is the most important thing.

★ There is much more to people than just what they look like.

What do we think about girls and boys?

❶ Describe what you think about:

Boys' toys	Girls' toys
Girls when they play together	**Boys when they play together**
How girls behave in lessons	**How boys behave in lessons**
What boys must never do or people might laugh at them	**What girls must never do or people might laugh at them**

❷ Underline anything you have written that you do not think is a particularly good thing.

❸ Do boys and girls see anything differently?

Activity sheet 3 * SRE 7–9 © Molly Potter 2009

Family

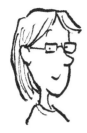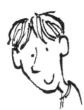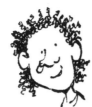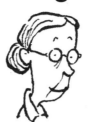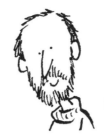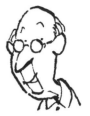

A lot of families could be described as a group of people related to each other by blood or marriage, or a group of people who live in the same home. However, not all families follow the pattern of having a married mother and father living together with their children – like you often see in storybooks.

Here are some ways in which families can be different:

★ They can be large (with lots of children) or small.

★ There might be only one adult in the family – a mum, a dad or a carer.

★ Not all mums and dads are married – some just live together.

★ Some children live with their carers.

★ Some children have been adopted.

★ Some children live with their mother/father and their mother's girlfriend/father's boyfriend.

★ Some children's mothers and/or fathers have married more than once and their children live with their stepmother or stepfather and possibly stepbrothers and stepsisters as well.

★ Some children live with their grandparents.

People expect members of a family to be close and to love one another – whoever it is that makes up that family. Some families are very close and get on with each other all the time. However, an old saying says that 'you can choose your friends but you can't choose your family'. People in the same family can experience problems with each other.

In pairs, discuss the following things:

❶ What is good about belonging to a family?

❷ What kind of things do parents and carers do for their children?

❸ What kind of things do families do together?

❹ Is it better to be the older or the younger child in a family?

❺ What do you think is good about being an only child, or having brothers or sisters?

❻ If you were to write a list of rules for parents and carers, what would you include in your list?

（57）

Appendices

An example pre-programme letter
(page 59)

This can be sent to parents and carers prior to embarking upon an SRE programme. It gives a brief outline of the programme, reminds parents/carers of their right to withdraw their child, states what is statutory in the Science National Curriculum and invites them to contact the school if they have any concerns.

Sex and Relationship Education (SRE) information for parents/carers
(pages 60-61)

This can be used to inform parents/carers about SRE and to address their commonly cited concerns.

Parents'/carers' consultation form
(page 62)

This can be used to ascertain parents'/carers' views about SRE. It is considered good practice to do some kind of consultation with parents/carers about SRE prior to the review or instigation of an SRE programme. Generally, schools find that when they involve parents/carers in this way, there are many advantages:

★ It puts SRE on everyone's agenda.
★ It makes parents/carers feel valued for their input.
★ It usually helps the school to realise that the vast majority of parents/carers are supportive of SRE.
★ It highlights any particular concerns parents/carers might have that the school might not have considered.
★ It goes part way to addressing criteria on the school's Self-evaluation Form (SEF).
★ Nearly always, after an appropriately led consultation, the views of most uncertain parents/carers have shifted to a more 'liberal' position.

It needs to be noted that parents/carers do not have a legal right to vote for what is and is not included in a school's SRE programme. Their ultimate legal right, however, is to withdraw their child from the programme. If a parent/carer chooses to exercise this right, it is best that they do so and the programme is still accessible to the majority of pupils.

Pupils' consultation form (SRE) (page 64)

This can be used to ascertain pupils' views about SRE. It is excellent practice to take pupils' views about SRE into consideration. Consultation with them often shows that they have picked up the embarrassment felt around these issues in the UK (this can be addressed through ground rules) and often highlights that pupils have considered SRE-related issues more than the adults in their lives might think. This can help to justify any programme you finally agree to deliver.

An example pre-programme letter

Dear Parent/Carer,

YEAR 4 SEX AND RELATIONSHIP EDUCATION (SRE) PROGRAMME

Over the next half a term, we will be running our six-week Sex and Relationship Education programme for Year 4 pupils. Below is an outline of the topics we will be covering:

- an introduction to the physical changes of puberty – including menstruation and sperm production;
- the emotional changes of puberty;
- how a baby is made;
- pregnancy and birth;
- a look at self-image and how the media affects us.

If you have any concerns or worries about the programme, or if you wish to discuss any aspect of it, please do not hesitate to contact the school.

YOUR RIGHT TO WITHDRAW YOUR CHILD FROM SRE LESSONS

As a parent/carer, you have a legal right to withdraw your child from the non-statutory SRE lessons (those that do not fall within the Science National Curriculum). If we do not hear from you, we will assume that you are willing for your child to take part in this programme.

FOR YOUR INFORMATION
Statutory at Key Stage 2 (Science National Curriculum):

Pupils should be taught:

- that the life processes common to humans and other animals include nutrition, growth and reproduction.
- about the main stages of the human life cycle.

Sex and Relationship Education (SRE)

information for parents/carers

What is SRE?

Sex and Relationship Education is not just about teaching facts about sex and body matters, as these alone will have limited impact on the decisions young people may make. An effective SRE programme also aims to:

★ help children to develop life skills (such as resisting peer pressure, being assertive, making informed decisions, negotiating skills, learning to respect others, emotional intelligence etc.).

★ give pupils lots of opportunities to explore and develop their own and others' attitudes, values and opinions (for example, what makes something 'wrong'?).

What do we hope to achieve with an effective SRE programme?

An effective SRE programme will help pupils to develop:

★ self-worth and self-awareness;
★ the skills needed for successful relationships;
★ an understanding of their own and others' rights;
★ the ability to express how they feel about situations;
★ the ability and confidence to make informed choices;
★ the ability to keep themselves and other people safe;
★ an understanding of their own and others' values and beliefs, and an individual moral framework that will help them to make positive decisions;
★ a discerning eye for the messages they receive from the media;
★ a positive attitude towards the way people can be different from each other;
★ a positive attitude towards their own bodies;
★ the ability and confidence to access help and support.

Why do we need SRE at primary school?

We live in a society where, on the one hand, all matters relating to sex are often not spoken about and, on the other, children are bombarded with images of suggested sex from a variety of sources e.g. TV, magazines, adverts, graffiti, the internet, friends, older children etc.. A big part of SRE is to help children to challenge the unrealistic and inaccurate messages they receive from some of these sources and the earlier this starts, the more effective it will be.

Covering SRE from an early age 'normalises' the subject and makes children feel more comfortable talking about issues that concern them. If children and young people become more at ease speaking about these matters, they are more likely to be responsible — as to be responsible about sex usually involves a conversation!

It is better to equip children with knowledge and skills before they need to draw upon them — the teenage years are usually not the best time to start discussions about sex and relationships. In fact, research has shown that this can be a very uncomfortable experience for many teenagers if they have had no conversations with their parents/carers about these matters when they were younger.

Often, when we reflect on our own school's SRE, we realise that it probably suffered in quality and quantity because of everyone's discomfort with the subject. Do we really want this to continue? When we consider SRE beyond a 'gut reaction' of discomfort, we often realise this response is not always a rational one. The UK's high teenage pregnancy rate and high incidence of sexually transmitted infections (STIs) show that our SRE has room for improvement!

Common concerns about SRE

Although SRE is not just delivering factual information about sexual matters, this is the part of SRE that causes the most anxiety. Frequently cited concerns are:

'Too much knowledge can be dangerous.'

Children often know and speculate about sex more than parents/carers probably suspect — some of it correct and some of it, at times, a little confused. Is knowledge alone actually dangerous? SRE aims to help pupils to make responsible use of any knowledge they gain. Research also shows that effective SRE does not encourage children to 'experiment'.

'Surely parents/carers are best placed to deliver SRE?'

Ideally — yes — but many parents/carers are not comfortable talking to their children about sex. For example, single parents sometimes highlight their uneasiness or lack of knowledge when it comes to talking about the opposite sex and are grateful that the school is doing this for them.

'Keep children innocent — do they really need to learn about sex? Can't we protect them?'

Parents and carers that teach their children how babies are made at an early age would certainly argue that their children are no less innocent for having this information. This knowledge does not appear to 'damage' children and furthermore they also pick up the message that adults are prepared to talk about these matters and can be asked for help. We will never be able to 'protect' our children always and forever — all we can do is equip them with information and skills and then trust them.

'How explicit will the programme be?'

Each individual school decides upon the content of its own SRE programme. Careful consideration is put into how detailed the programme needs to be and how to answer children's questions. Many parents/carers appreciate their children's questions being answered openly and honestly — but with discretion exercised over explicitness.

'Will what is taught go against my personal beliefs?'

SRE aims to enhance personal values of respect and acceptance. This means no single view is taught as the 'correct' view and pupils are encouraged to respect the fact that there is a diversity of views with most issues. In effective SRE, the teacher does not impose their personal views on the pupils and most issues are explored in terms of personal choice.

'They seem so young – are they really ready for all this?'

Puberty starts younger (as young as eight) these days and even now, 10% of girls in the UK start their periods without knowing what is happening to them. This can be extremely scary. Preparation for puberty at secondary school is too late.

Investigations into what pupils already know often reveal that they have picked up a lot of knowledge from the media and playground speculation at very young ages. It would be better for children to be given the correct knowledge from a sensitively taught and accurate school's programme than for children to fall prey to misunderstandings that can be quite distressing.

Last word...

Pupils might use the geography they learn at school and they might use the art, but they will definitely use what they learn in SRE!

For information on government guidance on schools' SRE, visit:

http://publications.dcsf.gov.uk/

Type in 'Sex and Relationship Education' guidance in the 'Online Publications' search box to take you to the relevant document.

Parents'/carers' consultation form

Sex and Relationship Education (SRE) – parents'/carers' information and questionnaire

Dear Parents/carers,

We are currently having a look at our school's Sex and Relationship Education policy and programme. We consider it very important that we ask parents and carers what they think about this topic before we make any decisions on what we are going to teach and how we are going to teach it.

If you would like your views to be considered, please complete the following questionnaire and return it to the school by _____.

SEX AND RELATIONSHIP EDUCATION – BACKGROUND INFORMATION

The only part of Sex and Relationship Education that the law tells schools they have to teach is found in the Science National Curriculum.

SRE parts of the Science National Curriculum:

Key Stage 1 (5–7 year olds)

Pupils should be taught:

- that animals, including humans, move, feed, grow, use their senses and reproduce.
- to recognise and compare the main external parts of the bodies of humans.
- that humans and animals can produce offspring and that these grow into adults.
- to recognise similarities and differences between themselves and others, and treat others with sensitivity.

Key Stage 2 (7–11 year olds)

Pupils should be taught:

- that the life processes common to humans and other animals include nutrition, growth and reproduction.
- about the main stages of the human life cycle.

The other parts of SRE are not compulsory, so each individual school has to decide upon what it is going to teach within PSHE (Personal, Health and Social Education).

SRE 7–9 * © Molly Potter 2009

Questionnaire

❶ Please indicate on this table the earliest age at which you think these three factual Sex and Relationship Education topics should be covered in a school's SRE programme. If you do not believe something should be covered, please cross it out, and if you think the topic should be left to a secondary school, please write S in the table.

TOPIC	Year group or age topic should first be taught
the physical and emotional changes of puberty	
sexual intercourse	
pregnancy and birth	

Do you have any comments about this table?

_____

_____

❷ Do you think the school should answer any question about sex that a child asks?   (Circle your answer.)   YES/NO

Please comment:

_____

_____

❸ How do you feel about some topics being taught in single-sex groups?

_____

_____

_____

❹ Every parent/carer has the right to remove their child from SRE lessons (other than the Science National Curriculum parts). Do you think, as a parent/carer, you would wish to remove your child? (Circle your answer.) Yes/No

Please comment:

_____

_____

❺ Do you have any worries about SRE? If so, please comment.

_____

_____

❻ Would you like to say anything else about this matter? Please use overleaf if needed.

_____

_____

Thank you for taking time to complete this form. We will consider your comments when we are making decisions about what to teach in SRE and how to teach it. You will be able to look at our draft policy and will be invited to make comments before we decide to finally use the policy.

All questionnaires will be treated confidentially. There is no need to add your name, but if you wish to, then please do so.

Pupils' consultation form (SRE)

Name: _____

Please use the back of the sheet if you need to write more for any of the questions.

❶ What do you think Sex and Relationship Education (SRE) is about? _____

❷ Do you feel you know a lot of information about sex? (Please tick)

Yes, I do ☐   I know a fair bit ☐   There are lots of things about sex I don't know ☐   No, I don't feel I know much at all ☐

❸ At what age do you think you should first learn about the following things?

	Age
How babies are made	
What changes happen to your body as you grow up	

❹ What kind of things do you think you need to learn about in SRE? _____

❺ What do you think makes a good SRE teacher? _____

❻ Other than school, where else have you learnt about sex and relationships? Please tick.

Parents/carers		Any other sources of information? Please write here.
Friends		
Magazines		
Television		
Older brothers or sisters		

❼ Why do you think it's important for children to learn about sex and relationships at school? _____
_____

❽ Apart from your teachers, who else would you like to talk to about sex and relationships? _____

❾ Is there anything about SRE lessons that might worry you? If so, please comment. _____

❿ When you become a teenager, what kind of things to do with sex and relationships do you think you might worry about?
_____

⓫ Would you like it if the school staff were prepared to answer absolutely any question that you had about sex and relationships? (Please circle.) YES/NO
Why? _____

⓬ Would you like some SRE lessons to be taught to girls and boys separately? (Please circle.) YES /NO
Why? _____

⓭ Is there anything else you would like to say about SRE lessons? _____

SRE 7–9 * © Molly Potter 2009